Gerontological Nurse Practitioner Certification Review

D1452247

About the Authors

Meredith Wallace Kazer, PhD, APRN, A/GNP-BC, is Associate Professor, Fairfield University, School of Nursing. Dr. Kazer earned an MSN in medical–surgical nursing with a specialty in geriatrics from Yale University and a PhD in nursing research and theory development at New York University, where she won a predoctoral fellowship, Hartford Institute for Geriatric Nursing. In this capacity, she authored and edited the book series, *Try This: Best Practices in Geriatric Nursing*. In 2001, she won the Springer Publishing Company Award for *Applied Nursing Research*. She was the Managing Editor of the *Journal of Applied Nursing Research* and is currently the research brief editor for the journal. Dr. Kazer has also authored numerous journal articles and book chapters. At Springer, she published *Prostate Cancer: Nursing Assessment Management and Care (2002)*, an AJN Book of the Year Award winner; *Essentials of Gerontological Nursing (2007)*; *Gerontological Nurse Certification Review (2008)*, and acted as Associate Editor on another AJN Book of the Year Award winner, *Encyclopedia of Nursing Research*, 2nd edition (2006). In 2002, she was Associate Editor, *The Geriatric Nursing Research Digest*. She is a recent recipient of the ENRS/John A. Hartford Foundation investigator award. She is an adult and Gerontological Nurse Practitioner and currently practices in primary care with a focus on chronic illness in the elderly.

Sheila Grossman, PhD, APRN, FNP-BC, is a Professor of Nursing and Coordinator of the Family Nurse Practitioner Track at Fairfield University School of Nursing. She received a BS in nursing from the University of Connecticut, her MS as a Respiratory Clinical Nurse Specialist from the University of Massachusetts Amherst, a postmaster's degree as a Family Nurse Practitioner from Fairfield University, and her PhD from the University of Connecticut. She has worked for many years as a clinician on a variety of medical, surgical, and critical care units and presently practices as a Family Nurse Practitioner in a primary care clinic. She is the coauthor of *The New Leadership Challenge: Creating a Preferred Future for Nursing*, which is in its third edition (2009), and received an AJN Book of the Year Award and has also received an AJN Book of the Year Award for *Mentoring in Nursing: A Dynamic and Collaborative Process (2007)*, and coauthored *Gerontological Nurse Certification Review* in 2008 with Dr. Meredith Wallace Kazer. She is the author of multiple chapters and journal articles on leadership, mentoring, gerontology, adult health, and palliative care. Her research interests focus on symptom management in palliative care, leadership, pedagogy, cultural competence, and adult patient outcome studies. She is active in Sigma Theta Tau International Honor Society, American Association of Critical Care Nurses, National Organization of Nurse Practitioner Faculty, and American College of Nurse Practitioners and is a certified End of Life Nursing Education Consortium Educator and a Commission on Collegiate Nursing Education Accreditation Site Visitor. She is the winner of the 2009 Josephine Dolan Award for Outstanding Contributions to Nursing Education sponsored by the CT Nurses Association.

Gerontological Nurse Practitioner Certification Review

Meredith Wallace Kazer, PhD, APRN, A/GNP-BC

Sheila Grossman, PhD, APRN, FNP-BC

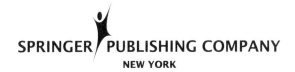

SPRINGER PUBLISHING COMPANY
NEW YORK

Springer Publishing Company, LLC
11 West 42nd Street
New York, NY 10036
www.springerpub.com

Acquisitions Editor: Allan Graubard
Senior Poduction Editor: Diane Davis
Cover Design: David Levy
Composition: S4Carlisle Publishing Services

ISBN 978-0-8261-0643-8
E-book ISBN: 978-0-8261-0644-5

11 12 13 14/ 5 4 3 2 1

The author and the publisher of this work have made every effort to use sources believed to be reliable to provide information that is accurate and compatible with the standards generally accepted at the time of publication. Because medical science is continually advancing, our knowledge base continues to expand. Therefore, as new information becomes available, changes in procedures become necessary. We recommend that the reader always consult current research and specific institutional policies before performing any clinical procedure. The author and publisher shall not be liable for any special, consequential, or exemplary damages resulting, in whole or in part, from the readers' use of, or reliance on, the information contained in this book. The publisher has no responsibility for the persistence or accuracy of URLs for external or third-party Internet Web sites referred to in this publication and does not guarantee that any content on such Web sites is, or will remain, accurate or appropriate.

Library of Congress Cataloging-in-Publication Data

Kazer, Meredith Wallace, PhD, RN.
  Gerontological nurse practitioner certification review / Meredith Wallace Kazer, Sheila Grossman.
    p. ; cm.
  Includes bibliographical references.
  ISBN 978-0-8261-0643-8
  1. Geriatric nursing—Examinations, questions, etc.   2. Nurse practitioners—Examinations, questions, etc.
I. Grossman, Sheila.   II. Title.
  [DNLM: 1. Geriatric Nursing—Examination Questions.   2. Nurse Practitioners—Examination Questions. WY 18.2]
  RC954.K39 2011
  618.97'0231—dc22

                                                                                        2010049721

Printed in the United States of America by Hamilton Printing.

To all of the nurse practitioners and nurse practitioner students we have collaborated with over the years. We also recognize the multiple older adult patients and their families we have enjoyed working with throughout our careers.

Meredith Wallace Kazer
Sheila C. Grossman

Contents

Foreword

With the large number of "baby boomers" who will begin to turn 65 years of age in 2011 and the tremendous advances in pharmaceutical, biotechnology, genetics, and other related sciences, we will see the largest number of the oldest of the old in the years to come. Today, people older than 75 years make up a smaller percentage of the population than do baby boomers. However, they use three or four times the number of hospital days as the boomers do. In addition, they use twice as many physician visits. If the trend continues, it will drive the cost of future health spending as the number of people 75 years old and older begins to grow.

Nursing is poised to have a tremendous impact on the quality and cost of care provided to this aging population. Through innovative models and evidence-based practice, nurses can define the care of the older person and avoid practices that lead to adverse or "never" events, such as restraints, inappropriate medication doses, change of medication regimen, failure to hydrate and provide adequate nutrition, and failure to provide appropriate skin care. Nurses with knowledge in geriatrics know that caring for an older person presents different challenges and requires age-specific protocols to meet the standards of quality, cost-effective care. The passage of the Health Reform Act will create a greater need for this kind of care.

Unfortunately, there are simply not enough health care providers in this country with the knowledge to address the needs of this growing segment of our population—older adults. There needs to be a sense of urgency to develop practitioners who can help patients avoid "never" events, prevent avoidable hospitalizations, and live lives at the fullest level of function and cognition possible. This requires consistent, collaborative, and coordinated care across the continuum. Many hospitals have more than half of their beds filled with older patients, and community-based care is most often provided to older adults. Nurses prepared in geriatrics can be the lynch pin in this process.

With a sense of commitment to have a significant impact on the health and well-being of our older population, the John A. Hartford Foundation has funded several initiatives to increase the capacity of the nursing profession to provide this evidence-based specialized care to older people. Increasingly, validation of specialized practice is through the certification process. This important new text is an important reference for nurses seeking to take the certification exam to validate their own practice. The practice of nursing over the next decades will demand age-specific knowledge for people across the life span. Nurses need to develop expertise in the area of geriatrics and have that expertise validated through certification.

Tara A. Cortes, PhD, RN, FAAN
Executive Director
The Hartford Institute for
Geriatric Nursing and
The Mathy D. Mezey Professor
in Geriatric Nursing

Preface

Gerontological Nurse Practitioner Certification Review will assist the reader in preparing for the American Nurses Credentialing Center and the American Academy of Nurse Practitioners Gerontological Nurse Practitioner (GNP) certification examinations. Additionally, it will help students in Gerontological Nurse Practitioner, Family Nurse Practitioner, and Adult Nurse Practitioner programs with their course program examinations that refer to older adults. The book was developed to review content specific to all GNP Competencies.

Chapter 1, *Information for Taking the Certification Exam*, describes all the information needed to sign up for the GNP exam, as well as the various details of applying for the GNP certification and Advanced Practice Registered Nurse (APRN) license. Chapter 2, *Question Analysis*, gives examples of how to read a question stem, review the potential answers, and identify the most appropriate answer. Examples of different types of questions that one can expect to see on the certification exam are explained. Chapter 3, *Health Promotion and Disease Prevention*, reviews Health People 2010–2020 in terms of older adults, along with specific information regarding their nutrition, exercise, and health screening. Chapter 4, *Assessment of Acute and Chronic Illness*, presents history and physical exam considerations, normal physiological aging changes, theories of aging, atypical presentations of illness, developmental changes, sexual function and well being, and diagnostic tests commonly used with older adults. Chapter 5, *Clinical Management of Older Adults*, reviews the pathophysiology and management for the most commonly seen disorders with older adults in each system. This chapter offers a longer chapter test because the certification examination is made up of more questions related to this material. Chapter 6, *Nurse Practitioner Role and Nurse–Patient Relationship*, reviews the role and scope, family involvement, teaching–coaching, and health literacy issues related to older adults. It also covers special issues such as palliative care, advanced directives, cultural awareness, elder abuse/neglect, driving, and health care disparities among the elderly. Chapter 7, *Health Care Systems and Policy*, discusses significant information related to older adults and the health care delivery system, health care policy, safety and the Institute of Medicine regarding Aging in America, quality improvement/outcome management, reimbursement, the Older American Act/OBRA, social security, Medicare and medigap, Medicaid, and long-term care insurance. The final chapter, Chapter 8, *Research Utilization*, describes utilization review, evidence-based practice, research, and ethical and legal issues related to older adults.

Each of these chapters has test questions at the end, which students should do as they complete each chapter. In addition, there is a test of 165 questions designed to offer the reader an opportunity to take a "mock test" of the Gerontological Nurse Practitioner Certification Exam after finishing the entire book. Answers for the test and chapter questions are provided at the end of the book. The reader should review all incorrectly answered questions with the text and then retake either the entire test or at least the questions that were not answered correctly the first time. This experience will assist the reader in being confidently prepared for the "real" certification exam. It is advised that the "mock test" be taken at least 3 weeks before the authentic exam date so that the reader will have adequate time to review the necessary material completely before the test date.

The authors hope those individuals using this review book will be productive and find the questions challenging and reflective of the authentic certification examinations.

Gerontological Nurse Practitioner Certification Review

1

Information for Taking the Certification Exam

This *Gerontological Nurse Practitioner Certification (GNP) Review* book prepares registered nurses (RNs) who have completed the necessary requirements to take the national Gerontological Nurse Practitioner Certification exam offered by the American Nurses Credentialing Center (ANCC) and the American Academy of Nurse Practitioners (AANP). By obtaining certification as a GNP, nurses gain power similar to that of board-certified physicians and other advanced practice nurses to function in a number of roles. GNPs are employed in primary care, long-term care, acute care, and other settings in which older adults live and visit. The ANCC defines GNPs as follows:

> The Gerontological Nurse Practitioner (GNP) is a registered nurse prepared in a graduate level gerontological nurse practitioner program to provide a full range of health care services on the wellness-illness health care continuum at an advanced level to older adults. The GNP practice includes independent and interdependent decision making and is directly accountable for clinical judgments. The graduate level preparation expands the GNP's role to include differential diagnosis and disease management, participation in and use of research, development and implementation of health policy, leadership, education, case management, and consultation. (*http://www.nursecredentialing.org/Eligibility/ GerontologicalNPEligibility.aspx*)

The need for GNPs is substantial given the rapidly increasing older adult population. At the onset of the 20th century, older adults made up only 4% of the U.S. population (3.1 million individuals). By mid-century, this number had grown to 12.3 million older adults or approximately 8% of the population (Rice & Fineman, 2004). Growth in the older adult population will continue to increase as the "baby boomers" turn 65 years of age beginning in 2011. By 2030, it is projected that 19% of Americans will be older than age 65 (http://www.aoa.gov/AoARoot/Aging_Statistics/index.aspx).

Qualified GNP candidates should be commended for positioning themselves to care for the growing population of older adults. Certification is an excellent way to be recognized for expertise in a specialty area and essential for licensing as advanced practice registered nurses (APRN) in most states.

The purpose of this chapter is to explain the following:

- The testing format

- The application and scheduling of the test date for certification

- General hints to improve your preparation for the exam.

Certification Exam Format

The ANCC and AANP offer only a computer-based test in multiple-choice format with the option of choosing one of four possible answers. The ANCC test contains 175 questions and covers content knowledge and application of professional nursing regarding gerontology at an entry-level competency. The exam is developed from information from role delineation studies that measure the necessary knowledge and skills needed for competent practice in a specialty area such as gerontology (Stromberg et al., 2005). The purpose of the exam is to assess whether nurses are competent to assess the strengths of older adults to facilitate their highest quality of life and, when appropriate, a "good death." The ANCC updates the Gerontological Nurse Practitioner Certification exam on a regular basis. A 20-question practice certification examination and answers can be accessed at *http://test.nursecredentialing.org/GeroNP-Mar2010Test.htm*. Completing the practice exam and reviewing your answers is strongly recommended.

The examination topic areas focus on foundations of advanced practice, advanced assessment, and advanced management. Questions will also be asked on advanced nursing ethics, policy, leadership and research. The additional questions are pilot test questions and may fall into any of these three categories.

Detailed Test Content Outline

This book is designed to prepare students to answer the questions in the ANCC and AANP GNP test content outlines (which can be seen in detail at *http://www.nursecredentialing.org/Documents/Certification/TestContentOutlines/*

GerontologicalNPMar2010.aspx or *https://www.aanpcertification.org/ptistore/control/certs/domains*).

TOTAL NUMBER OF QUESTIONS

There are 175 questions on the ANCC test, but 25 of them are pilot questions and do not count toward one's score. There is no way to determine which of the 175 questions count for your test, so it is best to consider each question as carefully as you can. This is the standard approach for validating new questions and ensuring that they are reliable.

TOTAL TIME

The time allowed to take the ANCC test is 3.5 hours. If desired, test takers can take a 20-minute practice exam to become oriented to the computer system, before the start of the examination. This is highly recommended for all test takers. Most people complete the exam in about 2.5 hours, but ANCC allows 3.5 hours to take the exam.

Obtaining the Application

ELIGIBILITY TO TAKE THE EXAM

To qualify for the examination, ANCC and AANP requires the following:

- Hold a current, active RN license in a state or territory of the United States or the professional, legally recognized equivalent in another country.

- Hold a master's, post-master, or doctorate degree from a GNP program accredited by the Commission on the Collegiate of Nursing Education (CCNE) or the National League for Nursing Accrediting Commission (NLNAC). A minimum of 500 faculty supervised clinical hours must be included in your GNP program. The GNP graduate program must include course work in advanced health assessment, advanced pharmacology, advanced pathophysiology, health promotion and disease prevention, differential diagnosis, and disease management.

In addition to the traditional educational program track toward GNP certification, an alternative route to certification is available for an undetermined period of time. This alternative eligibility route to GNP certification is available as a secondary certification only to currently certified and licensed acute care nurse practitioners, adult nurse practitioners, or family nurse practitioners.

This alternative eligibility is available to increase the number of practicing GNPs to fill the care needs of the increasing older adult population as described earlier. It is important to note that the ANCC indicates that this secondary certification may not be recognized by all state boards of nursing. Thus, it is important to contact your state board of nursing before taking this secondary examination to determine if it is recognized by your state. Candidates interested in obtaining certification via this alternative route must meet the eligibility criteria as stated by the ANCC (which is available at *http:// www.nursecredentialing.org/Eligibility/GerontologicalNPEligibility.aspx*).

Application

A *General Testing and Renewal Handbook* with testing information and an application can be accessed at *http://www.nursecredentialing.org/Documents/ Certification/Application/NursingSpecialty/GerontologicalNursePractitioner .aspx* or *https://www.aanpcertification.org/ptistore/resource/documents/ GERO_APP_2009.pdf* or *https://www.aanpcertification.org/ptistore/control/ certs/process* (AANP, 2010).

If you have any questions regarding the application, you can send an e-mail to A certification@ana.org or call 1-800-284-2378, or AANP at certification@ aanp.org or call (512) 442-5202.

Scheduling the Test

Once you submit the application and are approved to take the examination, you will receive notification via mail with instructions on how to schedule the examination. This authorization to test (ATT) will be mailed to you from ANCC. After you receive the ATT, call 1-800-350-7076 or visit *http://www.2test.com* and make an appointment during the 90-day eligibility time period stated on your ATT form. The test is administered by Thomson Prometric Computer Testing Centers. To choose a location, first set up a date and time to take the computerized test on Prometric's Web site (*http:// securereg3.prometric.com*).

Testing centers are located in every state in the United States and some sites in Canada, Puerto Rico, and Guam. You can schedule, reschedule, or cancel your appointment at the Prometric Web site (*http://www.2test.com*). Hours for testing are generally 8:00 A.M. to 5:00 P.M., and the testing centers are open Monday through Friday. It is recommended that you schedule your test appointment as soon as you get your ATT in order to have the best opportunity of getting your desired day and time. If you decide to switch the date, time, or test site location, you need to follow the directions in the ANCC or AANP application instructions. A fee may apply for rescheduling.

What to Bring on the Day of the Exam

You need to bring your ATT form and two forms of identification that match the name on your ATT. One form of ID must have your photo, and both forms must have your signature. One form must be your passport, a photo driver's license, or a photo government-issued ID card. You will not be admitted without the necessary forms of identification. You cannot take anything into the testing room. You will be provided with scratch paper and a pencil only. You will be given a locker to store your valuables, such as car keys and wallet.

Time of Arrival

Test takers must arrive 15 minutes earlier than the scheduled time. Failure to arrive early will cost you your appointment and require you to reapply.

During the Exam

There are no refreshment breaks. You can take a restroom break according to the instructions given at the testing center, but this time will be subtracted from your total time. You cannot ask any questions during the exam. When you complete the test, you cannot take the scratch paper from the testing room.

Receiving Test Results

You will know whether you pass or fail the examination immediately after taking it. The results will be in a standardized format with a pass or fail designation. Those who fail the exam will receive a diagnostic explanation for each of the content areas.

Receiving Certificate and Pin

Those who pass the exam receive a certificate, pin, and identification card that states ANCC or AANP certification by mail, following the examination. This certification is valid for 5 years. Information regarding recertification is available at *http://www.nursecredentialing.org* or *https://www.aanpcertification.org/ptistore/control/recert/recert_docs*

Hints for the Certification Exam

- There is no penalty for guessing, so it is recommended that test takers answer every question.

- There is an option to mark questions that you are not sure of and return to them later. This is a good idea, as other questions may give you clues to the answers you are unsure of.

- The test covers general and advanced gerontological problems, not rare and exotic diseases; some of the diseases to focus and study on include iron and chronic illness anemia, congestive heart failure, hypertension, diabetes, common skin lesions, postherpatic neuralgia, osteoporosis, polymyalgia rheumatica, and pressure ulcers.

- Be familiar with the common drugs used with older adults and their therapeutic levels.

- Know the frequently occurring adverse drug events with older adults and be able to apply the Modified Beers Criteria.

- You should know the normal laboratory results for the diseases that older adults commonly experience.

- There is a strong focus on health promotion guidelines, such as exercise and immunization recommendations.

- GNPs must also know Medicare, Medicaid, and other major insurance eligibility criteria and reimbursement guidelines.

References that are recommended by the ANCC regarding gerontology are available at *http://www.nursecredentialing.org/TestReferences/GerontologicalNP Mar2010.aspx*

REFERENCES

Rice, D. P., & Fineman, N. (2004). Economic implications of increased longevity in the United States. *Annual Review of Public Health, 25,* 457–473. UC San Francisco. Retrieved from http://escholarship.org/uc/item/4912f66t

Stromberg, M., Niebur, B., Prevost, S., Fabrey, L., Muenzen, P., Spence, C., et al. (2005). Specialty certification, more than a title. *Nursing Management, 5*(5), 36–40.

U.S. Department of Health and Human Services. (2003). *Health, United States, 2003.* Hyattsville, MD. Washington, DC: U. S. Government Printing Office.

2

Question Analysis

Preparing for a standardized exam often causes anxiety and fear in individuals. There are a number of strategies that examination takers may use to lessen these fears and anxieties and also help to prepare for the exam. It is important to remember that to meet the eligibility criteria for the exam, you would have had to complete an educational program to prepare you for the exam, or in the case of alternative eligibility, you have years of experience as a nurse practitioner. Regardless of the path taken to bring you to the test, you possess both knowledge and experiences that will serve as excellent resources while preparing for the Gerontological Nurse Practitioner (GNP) examination. As an adult, you also have life experience and either preceptored and/or independent experiences with the nursing process in multiple situations with older adults that have prepared you for:

- Assessing

- Analyzing situations and prioritizing

- Planning

- Implementing the plan of care

- Evaluating patient outcomes.

Experience with the nursing process trains the brain to clinically analyze practice situations, which will assist greatly in analyzing examination questions. Questions on the examination fall into a number of categories of the nursing process. Some questions require assessment expertise. Other questions require examination takers to prioritize care. Still other questions require the development of a treatment plan for a specific patient outcome, given the data presented in the question. Other questions require examination

TABLE 2.1

Performance in Clinical Practice Mirrors Thought Processes for Taking the Gerontological Nurse Practitioner Exam

Clinical Practice	Analyzing Examination Question
Assess the patient with comprehensive review of symptoms during admission or episodically.	Take the data significant for assessment of the patient from the stem and match these with what the point of the question is.
Analyze all the data you collected in assessment and use them to plan the patient's care.	Take the significant clues assessed from the question stem and prioritize all the information so that you can make the most appropriate plan.
Plan the treatment necessary to care appropriately for the patient's needs. Remember to make priorities.	Review the stem of the question and choose the information that tells you the patient's diagnosis, current status, and if there is any priority situation that needs immediate attention. Analyze this together, and select from the possible answers the plan that best fits the patient's needs.
Implement the plan with a possible need for rescheduling some actions given the patient's needs.	Take the significant clues in the stem of the question that indicate what the patient needs now and in the future. Analyze all the information and choose the sequence of actions that you would follow if this were your patient in practice.
Evaluate your patient's outcomes with respect to the appropriate plan that was implemented.	Review the stem of the question and brainstorm what exactly you would be evaluating, given the diagnosis and patient status. Choose the answer based on the standards of care and evidence-based practice you follow in clinical practice.

takers to choose appropriate methods of evaluating a clinical situation, given a particular set of data. Regardless of the way the question is interpreted, you will be critically thinking through the scenario using the nursing process. Your thought processes will mirror what you would have done with similar situations if you were at your work setting. Table 2.1 outlines the similar thought processes used when taking the exam or being in practice.

10 Test-Taking Strategies

Regardless of your preparation for the GNP examination, a number of test-taking strategies may be useful to you in choosing the correct answers on the examination. It is important to identify that there are two parts in each question. The sentence or phrase that follows the question number is called the stem. The four possible answers are called distracters, although only one of these is a correct answer. The following strategies will help to analyze the stem and distracters effectively:

1. Read the question stem carefully. There will be some essential information in the question that should be noted as well as some information that is irrelevant. Use the paper and pencil provided to make note of the essential information in the question. What is the essential information in the following question?

   A 93-year-old female complains of nausea, sweating, and feeling "very weak" over the last 8 hours. She presents in the emergency department with a history of gastroesophageal reflux disease (GERD), coronary artery disease (CAD), and coronary artery bypass graph (CABG) within the last 3 months. She has no other complaints. After taking vital signs, which are stable, your next step in assessing this patient would be to

   A. Take a finger stick to assess blood sugar

   B. Perform an electrocardiogram (EKG)

   C. Draw bloods for chemistry profile, complete blood count (CBC) with differential

   D. Contact the geriatrician on call.

   Essential information in this question includes symptoms (nausea, sweating, and feeling "very weak"), diagnosis (GERD, CAD, and CABG) within the last 3 months, time since symptoms (8 hours), and actions already taken (vital signs stable). As all patients in the GNP examination are older adults, the age of the patients will not likely play a substantial role in the individual examination questions and could be considered not essential.

2. The next strategy is to determine the type of answer you are asked to select. Is the question asking for you to select the next step in assessment, a diagnostic test, diagnosis, or treatment option? What type of answer is the question asking the student to select? If you selected the next step in assessment, you are correct. With this information in mind, you know that any answers that do not provide assessment data (such as answer D) are incorrect.

3. After full analyses of the question, but before you look at the answer choices, use the paper and pen provided to write down what you believe the correct answer is. Many successful examination takers feel that it is good to cover the distracters with a piece of paper or one's hand and to read the stem of the question without looking at the distracters. Given your

academic preparation and clinical experience, you are likely to have an idea of the answer to the question. Writing it down before you review the answer choices will help you to choose between seemingly correct answer choices. After reading the stem, it is felt by many that the examination taker should reflect on the question stem and think what comes to mind as the answer. This process seems to be helpful to many successful examination takers.

4. Given your education and clinical experience, you may suspect answer A to be a good choice. Even though you have an answer in mind, be sure to read all answer choices. It is likely that there may be more than one answer that incorporates your idea of the correct response.

5. Once you have an answer in mind and have read all the answer choices, it is time to rule out incorrect answer choices. You may suspect that answers B and C are good choices in this question. However, would you draw blood before a simple blood sugar or EKG? Probably not, given the time it would take to return results. Given the patient's symptomatology, answer A (FBS) is more appropriate than answer B (EKG). Let's look at another question and employ all our examination strategies.

MN has been admitted to your unit with congestive heart failure (CHF). Which of the following symptoms are most likely to be present in this 93-year-old?

A. Cough

B. Decreased cognitive status

C. Fever

D. Sudden-onset pedal edema.

Essential information in this question includes the diagnosis (CHF). The name, gender, and age of this patient (except that she is an older adult) are irrelevant. The type of answer needed is to identify symptoms. Thus any answer options that are not symptoms can be eliminated. At this point, take a guess and write it down. Then read all answer options; is your answer there? Next eliminate incorrect answers. Your knowledge of normal changes of aging and CHF will likely easily assist you in eliminating answer choice C. (Fever response in older adults is variable and not usually associated with CHF). This leaves answers A, B, and D.

6. After ruling out incorrect answer choices, review the remaining answer choices to see if there are parts of the answer that make it less than a correct choice for the question. It is significant to understand how some answer options contain two phrases or thoughts. These options are really sentences with two distinct points. Generally, the two phrases are connected by "and"

or "but." Both of these phrases must be true to have this two-component answer option to be the correct one. One might jump at a longer answer option, but this does not mean that this answer is the best answer. In the question involving MN, answer D is a good example of incorrect information within a potentially correct answer. Although we may expect pedal edema among CHF patients, we also know that CHF may be insidious in the older adult population, who may also have some pedal edema at baseline. Thus, *sudden-onset* pedal edema would be unlikely in this 93-year-old patient. Thus, answer choice D can be eliminated.

7. The examination taker should realize that sometimes the correct answer to a question is not what the examination taker may think is the most appropriate answer to a question. The examination taker must assume that there is a "best" answer to each question even though it may not be what he or she may perceive to be the most appropriate answer. In the question involving MN, you may have written down JVD or adventitious lung sounds as your most likely symptom that this CHF patient would have. However, neither of those answer choices were presented. Thus, you must select based on the answer choices provided.

8. When you are down to two answer choices that seem to be correct, be sure to select the most grammatically correct and comprehensive answer choice. When examination writers prepare questions, the correct answer is the one that gets written first and gets most attention. Thus, it is likely that this will be the most grammatically correct and complete answer in terms of grammar and information. Given the two remaining answer strategies for the question, answer choice A (cough) does not tell us as much as answer choice B. Is it a dry cough or moist productive cough? Answer choice B is likely with older adults who experience acute illness and also tells us that her cognitive status has declined.

9. If you have employed all of the strategies above and still cannot identify the correct answer choice, mark the question for review and move on to the next question. This is a good strategy for several reasons. First, too much time spent on one question may leave you short of time for answering the rest of the questions. Secondly, information provided in subsequent questions may give you a clue as to how to answer this question. Thirdly, time and space allow for a fresh read and perspective on the question, which may allow for effective selection of the correct answer.

10. It must be said that employment of excellent examination-taking strategies does not replace adequate examination review and preparation. A strong understanding of the content on the examination not only gives the knowledge needed to correctly select answer choices but also gives

examination takers the confidence that the choice selected will be the correct one. The following sections discuss the examination content and tips for reviewing and memorizing necessary examination material.

Review Content of Frequent Conditions Experienced by Older Adults

The American Nurse Credentialing Center provides a comprehensive test outline (see Chapter 1) that may serve as a guideline for examination review. Within this test outline, you may find some significant content information necessary to competently care for the older adult, which reflects assessing, analyzing, planning, implementing, and evaluating patient outcomes of conditions that older adults most frequently experience. A number of content areas in the care of older adults are heavily emphasized on in the exam. Although these are discussed in detail in this book, examination takers should review these areas more carefully if they feel that they do not have a competent level of knowledge regarding these content areas:

- Anemia (iron deficiency, chronic illness, folate and pernicious anemias)
- Medication management of CHF
- Medication management of HTN
- Diet and exercise management of diabetes
- Common skin lesions
- Postherpetic neuralgia
- Immunization guidelines
- Diagnoses of osteoporosis (T-Scores)
- Recommended exercise guidelines
- Tetanus immunization guidelines
- Therapeutic medication levels
- Pressure ulcer staging
- Thyroid disorder symptoms
- Polymyalgia rheumatica
- Medicaid/Medicare eligibility/restrictions

Strategies for Analyzing the Questions

Practice in answering the questions and timing oneself will assist in preparing one to be successful on a standardized examination such as this certification exam. The following are some further examples of challenging questions that may require some extra attention and the effective use of examination-taking strategies to assist in selecting the correct answer. Some sample questions with analyses are also given. See how you do.

EXAMPLE 1

Question

You are performing an eye assessment of an 80-year-old client. Which of the following findings is considered abnormal?

Answer Choices

A. Loss of outer hair on the eyebrows because of a decrease in hair follicles

B. The presence of arcus senilus seen around the cornea

C. A decrease in tear production

D. Unequal pupillary constriction in response to light

Relevant Information

Eye assessment, abnormal findings

Irrelevant Information

The exact age is irrelevant, except for the fact that the client is an older adult.

Type of Answer Needed

Abnormal change of aging

Your Guess

_____

_____

Incorrect Answer(s)

Loss of eyebrow hair (A) is a common and normal change of aging.

Dubious Answer Choice(s)

You may not be sure whether a decrease in tear production is normal with aging (C) or whether arcus senilus (B) is normal.

Correct Answer

Answer D. Unequal pupillary constriction is always abnormal.

EXAMPLE 2

Question

You are interviewing for a geriatric nurse practitioner position that requires you to participate primarily in tertiary prevention activities. These activities are designed to

Answer Choices

A. Prevent disease before it occurs

B. Detect disease at an earlier, more treatable stage

C. Manage disease, so it does not get worse

D. Eradicate all disease from the nation

Relevant Information

Tertiary prevention activities

Irrelevant Information

The fact that you are interviewing for a job is irrelevant.

Type of Answer Needed

Definition

Your Guess

Incorrect Answer(s)

Eradicate disease from the nation (D) is not a level of prevention or health care activity.

Dubious Answer Choice(s)

You may not be sure whether prevent disease before it occurs (A) or detect disease at an earlier, more treatable stage (B) are primary, secondary, or tertiary prevention activities. However, their order gives you a clue.

Correct Answer

Answer C. Manage disease, so it does not get worse.

EXAMPLE 3

Question

A 79-year-old male patient is complaining of pain, for which he needs medication. All of the following normal changes of aging should be considered when administering the medication, *except*

Answer Choices

A. Decreased hydrogen/oxygen breakdown

B. Decreased absorption from gastrointestinal track

C. Decreased metabolism of medications

D. Decreased renal clearance

Relevant Information

Medication needed

Irrelevant Information

Age and sex of patient

Type of Answer Needed

Abnormal change of aging related to pharmacodynamics

Your Guess

_____

_____

Incorrect Answer(s)

Older adults have a decreased rate of absorption from the GI track (B), so this is a normal finding and definitely not the answer to the question.

Dubious Answer Choice(s)

You may not be sure whether decreased hydrogen/oxygen breakdown (A) or decreased metabolism of medications (C) or decreased renal clearance occurs with aging; because answer A has little to do with medication pharmacodynamics, it stands apart from the rest.

Correct Answer

Answer A. Decreased hydrogen/oxygen breakdown.

EXAMPLE 4

Question

A 77-year-old male presents to the emergency department in acute pain. He says that he has new-onset left leg pain and that his leg is really swollen with erythematous streaks. He is diagnosed with

Answer Choices

A. Gout

B. Rheumatoid arthritis

C. Cellulitis

D. Fibromyalgia

Relevant Information

New-onset leg pain, edema, and erythematous streaks

Irrelevant Information

Age and sex of patient and presentation to ED

Type of Answer Needed

Diagnosis

Your Guess

_____

_____

Incorrect Answer(s)

Answers (A) gout and (B) rheumatoid arthritis are both joint diseases and would rarely present as leg pain.

Dubious Answer Choice(s)

Fibromyalgia (D) symptoms are more vague but would not normally present with erythematous streaks.

Correct Answer

Answer C, Cellulitis.

EXAMPLE 5

Question

You are asked to participate in a research study. If a study is said to use a random sampling, this means the sample was

Answer Choices

A. Representative of the average American

B. Chosen on the basis of convenience

C. Determined using clustering technique to ensure homogeneity

D. Selected so that each member of a population has an equal probability of being included

Relevant Information

Random sampling

Irrelevant Information

You are asked to participate in a research study.

Type of Answer Needed

Definition

Your Guess

_____

_____

Incorrect Answer(s)

Answer B is the definition of convenience sampling, and answer C focuses on homogeneity, which is not consistent with the goal of random sampling.

Dubious Answer Choice(s)

Answer A, representative of the average American is not a bad answer or incorrect, but it is not a full or comprehensive definition of random sampling.

Correct Answer

Answer D. Selected so that each member of a population has an equal probability of being included.

Clues to Memorizing Information

It is helpful when reviewing content before taking an exam to have certain methods of remembering information. For example, everyone knows the three P's that indicate the three most frequent manifestations of diabetes mellitus—(1) polydipsia, extreme thirst; (2) polyuria, frequent urination; and (3) polyphagia, extreme hunger. Remembering this sequence will assist in answering the following question.

EXAMPLE 1

A 66-year-old individual shares with you that she is "eating like a cow" and "drinking everything in sight." She says that this has been going on over the last few months. You enquire if she has also had urinary frequency for which she responds "yes I have." As the nurse caring for her, you decide to call the attending physician to request

A. Increased calories with the diet

B. A nutritionist consultation

C. A fasting blood sugar for the next morning*

D. Stat blood work for an HgbA1C

Rationale for correct answer—C. The three P's are clearly spelled out by the patient and warn that she may be developing diabetes mellitus. The patient is not in danger of hypoglycemia or hyperglycemia given the symptoms she has reported; therefore, choosing answer C, a fasting blood sugar for the next morning, will be the most reliable answer. There is no sense changing the diet or getting the nutritionist involved until it is known whether she has diabetes mellitus or not. HgbA1C is not a diagnostic measurement.

EXAMPLE 2

A 77-year-old woman did not have an intact gag reflex in the neurological examination. The cranial nerve affected is

A. V

B. IX*

C. XI

D. X

Rationale for correct answer—B. This is pure recall, so you have to memorize it by applying the information to a framework that you can remember. The gag reflex is absent in patients with damage to the glossopharyngeal nerve, which is the IX cranial nerve as it is responsible for the afferent limb of the reflex. First, you need to remember the cranial nerve mnemonic to identify the 12 cranial nerves. Then you have to review what functions you have memorized for each cranial nerve. Using a mnemonic such as ***On Old Olympus' Towering Top A Finn And German Viewed Some Hops*** is very helpful and easily retained in your memory.

EXAMPLE 3

A 71-year-old woman has been taking steroids for her asthma for 25 years. She presents with increased weight and puffy ankles, states she feels hyperactive and "stressed," and complains "I have increased hair in all of the wrong places." She is most likely developing the following syndrome:

A. Addison's disease

B. Cushing's disease*

C. Hyperaldosteronism

D. Hypoaldosteronism

Rationale for the correct answer—B. The fact that this patient has been taking steroids for several years provides a good clue to the answer to the question. This together with a consistency of symptoms specific for Cushing's syndrome helps to rule out the other answers, leaving answer choice B.

Summary and Conclusions

To be successful at any examination, students must be familiar with the test content. However, even knowledgeable students may get nervous when taking examinations. Moreover, despite excellent preparation, students may not know answers to some questions. This chapter provides information on how to prepare for the GNP examination and strategies to analyze and answer questions to which the answers are known and those for which answers are not known. By reviewing these test-taking strategies, students will have the best possible chance at test success.

3

Health Promotion and Disease Prevention

Health promotion and disease prevention practices developed over the past several decades play a substantial role in the increased lifespan of older adults today. In 2003, the number of Americans aged 65 years and older was approximately 36 million or 12% of the population. By the year 2030, the percentage is projected to increase to more than 19% of the population (*http://www.aoa.gov/AoARoot/Aging_Statistics/index.aspx*). The fastest growing age group in the country is that of adults aged 85 years and older. It is anticipated that this population will continue to grow rapidly when the baby boomers, who begin to turn 65 on January 1, 2011, begin to move into this age group. According to Healthy People 2010, adults aged 65 years may be expected to live an average of 18 more years than they did 100 years ago, for a total of 83 years. Individuals aged 75 years can be expected to live an average of 11 more years, for a total of 86 years (USDHHS, 2000).

Although health promotion and disease prevention practices have been greatly enhanced over the past century, older adults may not have had access to such practices. The USDHHS reports that heart disease, cancer, and stroke continue to be leading causes of death among older adults, accounting for 63% of deaths in this population in the year 2000. Moreover, approximately 80% of older adults have at least one chronic medical illness, and 50% have at least two. These chronic medical illnesses have a direct connection with functional limitations among older adults. The most common chronic medical illness older adult live with are arthritis, hypertension, heart disease, diabetes, and obstructive lung diseases.

The causes of death and chronic illness among older adults are not always preventable. However, many of the risk factors for these diseases result from poor health practices. Despite their advanced age, older adults may still benefit from health promotion activities to decrease these risk factors even in their later years. In fact, health promotion is as important in older adulthood as it is in childhood. Older adults are never too old to improve their nutritional level, start exercising, get a better night's sleep, and improve their overall health and safety. The USDHHS developed Healthy People 2010: National Health-Promotion and Disease Prevention Objectives for health-promotion programs for the older population (USDHHS, 2001). These goals focus on increasing health-promotion programs and decreasing morbidity and mortality related to various disease states. The goals are currently being updated for a new document to be released soon entitled Healthy People 2020. Many of the goals of Healthy People 2010 and Healthy People 2020 focus on older adults. Exhibit 3.1 summarizes the new goals for older adults in Healthy People 2020.

This chapter reviews common health-promotion and disease-prevention strategies for older adults. The chapter begins with a discussion of barriers to common health-promotion activities for older adults. Then the chapter is organized by level of prevention. Primary prevention strategies are those that prevent a disease from occurring, such as immunizations and exercise. Secondary prevention activities detect diseases at an early treatable stage and may include common screening practices for older adults. Finally, tertiary

---

EXHIBIT 3.1 Objectives New to Healthy People 2020

- Reduce the proportion of older adults who have moderate to severe functional limitations.

- Reduce the proportion of unpaid caregivers of older adults who report an unmet need for caregiver support services.

- Increase the proportion of older adults with one or more chronic health conditions who report confidence in managing their conditions.

- Reduce the proportion of noninstitutionalized older adults with disabilities who have an unmet need for long-term services and supports.

- Reduce the rate of pressure ulcer-related hospitalizations among older adults.

- Increase the proportion of the health care workforce with geriatric certification.

- Increase the number of states and tribes that publicly report elder maltreatment and neglect.

- Increase the proportion of older adults with reduced physical or cognitive function who engage in light, moderate, or vigorous leisure-time physical activities.

- Reduce the rate of emergency department visits because of falls among older adults.

(Retrieved from *http://www.healthypeople.gov/hp2020/Objectives/TopicArea.aspx?id=37&TopicArea=Older+Adults*)

prevention strategies focus on disease management to prevent diseases from progressing and impacting morbidity and mortality.

Barriers to Health Promotion Among Older Adults

Health providers often hold misconceptions about the benefits of health promotion for older adults, thinking that older adults cannot benefit from these strategies. Moreover, separating the normal changes of aging from pathological illness makes it challenging to health care providers to set appropriate goals for health promotion.

Motivation to change in order to participate in health promotion activities is challenging among all age groups. Motivation is a key factor, especially in changing long-established and difficult health behaviors such as smoking, excessive alcohol use, poor nutritional habits, and sedentary life styles. Motivational theory is generally associated with workplace employment and the desire to develop more effective employees but may be applied to improving health behaviors. Frederick Herzberg's work is important in this area. Other key motivation theories include McGregor's X-Y theory, Adams' Equity theory, McClelland's Motivational theory, and Erikson's Psychosocial theory. Motivational theories support the notion that it is critical to determine the motivational factor to change behavior. Thus, the determination of a critical end result and continuous feedback toward that result are important factors to change health behaviors among older adults. Researchers in motivational theory have identified the following potential motivators:

- Desire to avoid negative result of behavior

- Achievement of a goal

- Recognition of activity

- Health behavior itself

- Responsibility

- Advancement or progress

- Personal growth

Health promotion activities may be centered on these potential motivators to enhance compliance and success.

It is important to note that although Medicare may reimburse providers for illness-related care, many primary prevention strategies such as smoking cessation programs and exercise classes are not reimbursable under current health insurance policies. Older adults on limited incomes may not be able to afford to participate in such preventative health practices.

Levels of Prevention

PRIMARY PREVENTION

Primary prevention involves measures to prevent an illness or disease from occurring and includes the following:

- Exercise
- Smoking cessation
- Limited alcohol consumption
- Good nutrition
- Adequate sleep
- Safe lifestyles
- Updated immunizations

EXERCISE

The role of regular exercise in promoting health and preventing disease cannot be sufficiently emphasized. Regular exercise results in a number of positive health outcomes for older adults including the following:

- Reduced constipation
- Improved sleep
- Lower blood pressure
- Lower cholesterol levels
- Improved digestion
- Weight loss
- Enhanced opportunities for socialization
- Improved pain control

■ Increased temperature control in response to environmental changes

■ Reduced risk of hypothermia

Despite the many benefits of exercise among older adults, the amount of exercise generally decreases as one ages. The American College of Sports Medicine (ACSM) in conjunction with the American Heart Association (AHA) provides recommendations for older adults to use in the development and maintenance of an exercise program, as shown in Exhibit 3.2.

Interventions to promote exercise include helping older adults to choose an exercise program that they enjoy and in which they are motivated to participate. Older adults should consult their health care provider before the onset or substantial change in an exercise program to ensure that they are safely able to meet the aerobic demands of such a program. Sample exercise programs include the following:

■ Walking

■ Aquacise

EXHIBIT 3.2 Exercise Guidelines for Adults Older Than Age 65

Basic recommendations from ACSM and AHA:

Do moderately intense aerobic exercise 30 minutes a day, 5 days a week

Or

Do vigorously intense aerobic exercise 20 minutes a day, 3 days a week

And

Do 8 to 10 strength-training exercises, 10 to 15 repetitions of each exercise 2 to 3 times per week

And

If you are at risk of falling, perform balance exercises

And

Have a physical activity plan.

Both aerobic and muscle-strengthening activities are critical for healthy aging. Moderate-intensity aerobic exercise means working hard at about level-six intensity on a scale of 10. You should still be able to carry on a conversation during exercise.

Reprinted with permission from the American College of Sports Medicine (ACSM) and The American Heart Association (AHA).

EXHIBIT 3.3 Tips for Meeting Exercise Guidelines

With busy work schedules, family obligations, and packed weekends, it can often be difficult to get the recommended amount of physical activities. Try the following tips for incorporating exercise into your life:

■ Do it in short bouts. Research shows that moderate-intensity physical activity can be accumulated throughout the day in 10-minute bouts, which can be just as effective as exercising for 30 minutes straight. This can be useful when trying to fit physical activity into a busy schedule.

■ Mix it up. Combinations of moderate- and vigorous-intensity physical activity can be used to meet the guidelines. For example, you can walk briskly for 30 minutes twice per week and jog at a higher intensity on two other days.

■ Set your schedule. Maybe it is easier for you to walk during your lunch hour, or perhaps hitting the pavement right after dinner is best for you. The key is to set aside specific days and times for exercise, making it just as much a regular part of your schedule as everything else.

■ The gym is not a necessity. It does not take an expensive gym membership to get the daily recommended amount of physical activities. A pair of athletic shoes and a little motivation are all you need to live a more active, healthier life.

■ Make it a family affair. Take your spouse, your children, or a friend with you during exercise to add some fun to your routine. This is also a good way to encourage your kids to be physically active and get them committed early to a lifetime of health.

Reprinted with permission from the American College of Sports Medicine (ACSM).

■ Strength training, and

■ Yoga

The ACSM and the AHA provide the tips for beginning and maintaining an exercise program for older adults as described in Exhibit 3.3.

ALCOHOL USE

Alcohol dependence or alcoholism has the potential for great consequences among older adults, including negative effects on the following:

■ Function

■ Cognition

■ Health, and

■ Quality of life

Alcohol use is difficult to assess among older adults, because:

- Symptoms of alcohol use among older adults include alteration in mental status and function, which may mimic the symptoms of delirium, dementia, or depression.

- Older adults are usually no longer in the workforce, where the daily performance failures that are common with alcohol usage are often detected.

- Health care providers often have misconceptions about the prevalence of alcoholism among older adults. They are not always aware of how common alcohol is among older adult clients and thus, do not readily assess for it.

Alcoholism is a greater problem for older adults because older adults are not able to physiologically detoxify and excrete alcohol as effectively as younger people. Assessment of alcohol use may be most effectively accomplished using an instrument, such as the **CAGE** questionnaire that follows:

- Have you ever tried to **C**ut down on your drinking?

- Do you become **A**nnoyed when others ask you about drinking?

- Do you ever feel **G**uilty about your drinking?

- Do you ever use alcohol in the morning, as an **E**ye-opener?

Older adults with alcohol problems who receive treatment are capable of achieving positive health outcomes. In fact, when older adults receive effective treatment for their alcoholism, their prognosis is much better than it is for their younger counterparts. When alcohol abuse is suspected among older adults, it is necessary to refer them immediately to an appropriate program for effective treatment—such as Alcoholics Anonymous and/or an in- or outpatient detoxification and treatment program. Special treatment considerations must be applied to older adults during acute alcohol withdrawal related to normal and pathological aging changes. Effective alcohol withdrawal with the use of benzodiazepines while consistently monitoring vital signs and physiological response is essential to safely detoxify the older adult and prepare him or her for lifelong treatment.

SMOKING

Cigarette smoking has multiple harmful effects on older adults, including, but not limited to, cardiovascular and respiratory disease and cancer. The current cohorts of older adults are among the first people who have potentially smoked throughout their entire adult lives. It is possible for older adults to experience the benefits of smoking cessation even in old age. It is important to note that older adults may be more motivated to quit smoking than their younger counterparts because they are likely to experience some of the damage that smoking has caused. There are more available interventions available today than health care providers have ever had in the past. Over-the-counter nicotine replacement products in the form of gum, patches, and lozenges as well as prescription medications such as Wellbutrin and Chantix are all new products to assist older adults with smoking cessation. Older adults are encouraged to choose a quit date and to fill prescriptions in advance of the quit date (Sarna, & Bialous, 2010). Psychosocial support programs are also essential to smoking cessation and should be researched before attempts to quit smoking. If older adults are not successful in quitting smoking, it is important to remind them that most people are not successful the first time, and another quit date should be planned.

NUTRITION AND HYDRATION

It is estimated that approximately 20% of older adult diets are inadequate. The many risk factors for poor nutrition among older adults include the following:

- Normal changes of aging place older adults at a higher risk for nutritional deficiencies.

- Pathological diseases

- Decreases in smell, vision, and taste and the high frequency of dental problems

- Lifelong eating habits, such as a diet high in fat and cholesterol

- Diminishing senses of taste and smell result in less desire to eat and may lead to malnutrition.

- Limited income

- Lack of transportation to purchase food, and

- Social isolation.

Nutritional recommendations are among the first line of therapy for many diseases of older adults including hypertension, diabetes, and high cholesterol. To provide effective nutritional interventions, accurate nutritional assessments are essential and may include the following:

- 24-hour recall

- Nutritional assessments (see Figure 3.1).

Signs and symptoms of malnutrition may be seen in low levels of energy, alterations in skin integrity, nail beds, and hair quality. Thus a full physical assessment with both subjective and objective data collection will provide good information to diagnosis malnutrition. Associated lab data that may be

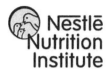

Mini Nutritional Assessment
MNA®

Last name:		First name:		
Sex:	Age:	Weight, kg:	Height, cm:	Date:

Complete the screen by filling in the boxes with the appropriate numbers. Total the numbers for the final screening score.

Screening

A Has food intake declined over the past 3 months due to loss of appetite, digestive problems, chewing or swallowing difficulties?
0 = severe decrease in food intake
1 = moderate decrease in food intake
2 = no decrease in food intake ☐

B Weight loss during the last 3 months
0 = weight loss greater than 3 kg (6.6 lbs)
1 = does not know
2 = weight loss between 1 and 3 kg (2.2 and 6.6 lbs)
3 = no weight loss ☐

C Mobility
0 = bed or chair bound
1 = able to get out of bed / chair but does not go out
2 = goes out ☐

D Has suffered psychological stress or acute disease in the past 3 months?
0 = yes   2 = no ☐

E Neuropsychological problems
0 = severe dementia or depression
1 = mild dementia
2 = no psychological problems ☐

F1 Body Mass Index (BMI) (weight in kg) / (height in m^2)
0 = BMI less than 19
1 = BMI 19 to less than 21
2 = BMI 21 to less than 23
3 = BMI 23 or greater ☐

IF BMI IS NOT AVAILABLE, REPLACE QUESTION F1 WITH QUESTION F2.
DO NOT ANSWER QUESTION F2 IF QUESTION F1 IS ALREADY COMPLETED.

F2 Calf circumference (CC) in cm
0 = CC less than 31
3 = CC 31 or greater ☐

Screening score ☐☐
(max. 14 points)

12-14 points: Normal nutritional status
8-11 points: At risk of malnutrition
0-7 points: Malnourished

For a more in-depth assessment, complete the full MNA® which is available at **www.mna-elderly.com**

Ref.   Vellas B, Villars H, Abellan G, et al. *Overview of the MNA® - Its History and Challenges.* J Nutr Health Aging 2006;10:456-465.
         Rubenstein LZ, Harker JO, Salva A, Guigoz Y, Vellas B. *Screening for Undernutrition in Geriatric Practice: Developing the Short-Form Mini Nutritional Assessment (MNA-SF).* J. Geront 2001;56A: M366-377.
         Guigoz Y. *The Mini-Nutritional Assessment (MNA®) Review of the Literature - What does it tell us?* J Nutr Health Aging 2006; 10:466-487.
         ® Société des Produits Nestlé, S.A., Vevey, Switzerland, Trademark Owners
         © Nestlé, 1994, Revision 2009. N67200 12/99 10M
         For more information: www.mna-elderly.com

FIGURE 3.1
Try this mini nutritional assessment

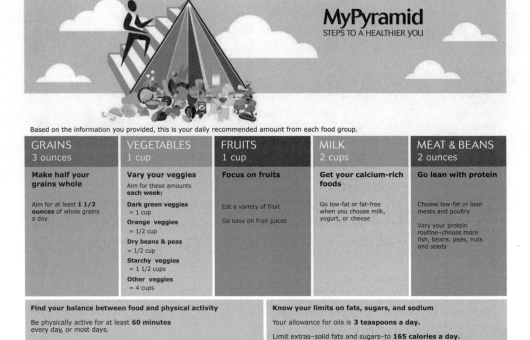

Based on the information you provided, this is your daily recommended amount from each food group.

GRAINS 3 ounces	VEGETABLES 1 cup	FRUITS 1 cup	MILK 2 cups	MEAT & BEANS 2 ounces
Make half your grains whole	**Vary your veggies** Aim for these amounts each week:	**Focus on fruits**	**Get your calcium-rich foods**	**Go lean with protein**
Aim for at least **1 1/2 ounces** of whole grains a day	**Dark green veggies** = 1 cup **Orange veggies** = 1/2 cup **Dry beans & peas** = 1/2 cup **Starchy veggies** = 1 1/2 cups **Other veggies** = 4 cups	Eat a variety of fruit Go easy on fruit juices	Go low-fat or fat-free when you choose milk, yogurt, or cheese	Choose low-fat or lean meats and poultry Vary your protein routine–choose more fish, beans, peas, nuts and seeds

Find your balance between food and physical activity	**Know your limits on fats, sugars, and sodium**
Be physically active for at least **60 minutes** every day, or most days.	Your allowance for oils is **3 teaspoons a day.** Limit extras–solid fats and sugars–to **165 calories a day.**

Your results are based on a 1000 calorie pattern   Name: _____

This calorie level is only an estimate of your needs. Monitor your body weight to see if you need to adjust your calorie intake.

FIGURE 3.2
Food guide pyramid
The U.S. Department of Agriculture *http://www.mypyramid.gov/downloads/results/results_1000_under9.pdf*

helpful include a prealbumin level, which will respond quickly to changes in protein intake.

Following nutritional assessments, teaching the patient regarding diets adequate in daily nutrients with limited intake of refined sugar and fats is recommended. A suggested resource is the MyPyramid food guide (see Figure 3.2). Periodic dietary assessments and reinforcements are needed to maintain adequate diets.

Failure to thrive (FTT) is a syndrome used to describe clients who experience malnutrition in the absence of an explanatory medical diagnosis. FTT is often found with the following:

- Dehydration

- Impaired cognition

- Dementia

- Impaired ambulation

- Difficulty with at least two activities of daily living, and

- Neglect.

SLEEP

The inability to fall asleep and to sleep through the night is among the most frequent complaints of older adults. Many older adults report difficulty falling asleep and frequent night-time awakenings. About half of older adults report one or more sleep problems. Key indicators of sleep disorders include the following:

■ Prolonged periods of difficulty falling asleep or getting back to sleep after night-time awakenings and

■ Daytime fatigue or sleepiness.

Sleep patterns are affected by both normal and pathological aging changes. The changes result in an increase in nocturnal awakenings, shorter periods of sleep, decrease REM sleep, and a decrease in slow-wave activity.

Sleep assessment is the first key to successful sleep management. It is important to note that while sleep medications may be helpful for short-term use, they are not indicated for long-term sleep management. Short-acting benzodiazepines should be selected, and all benzodiazepines should be used cautiously because of the possibility of rebound and morning insomnia, as well as hangover effect and daytime sedation (Frighetto et al., 2004). Nonpharmacological sleep interventions should be used whenever possible and may include the following:

■ Increase physical activity during the day.

■ Increase pain medication or alternative pain methods to help older adults suffering from painful conditions to get better rest at night.

■ Examine the sleep environment. Adjustments in noise and lighting may help older adults to sleep better.

■ Assess the stress in the lives of older adults. Identification and resolution of stressful life factors may help older adults to sleep more peacefully.

■ Daytime napping tends to interfere with a good night's sleep. Older adults who choose to nap during the day should acknowledge that the napping will likely reduce the total nighttime sleep needed.

ADULT IMMUNIZATION

One of the greatest advances in primary prevention and public health has been the use of immunizations to prevent disease. Adult immunization guidelines are provided in Figure 3.3.

Vaccine ▼ Age Group ►	19-26 Years	27-49 Years	50-59 Years	60-64 Years	≥65 Years
Tetanus, diphtheria, pertussis (Td/Tdap).*	Substitute one-time dose of Tdap for Td booster: then boost with Td every 10 years				Td booster every 10 years
Human papillomavirus.*	3 doses (females)				
Varicella.*	2 doses				
Zoster					1 dose
Measles, mumps, rubella.*	1 or 2 doses		1 dose		
Influenza.*			1 dose annually		
Pneumococcal (polysaccharide)	1 or 2 doses				1 dose
Hepatitis A.*	2 doses				
Hepatitis B.*	3 doses				
Meningococcal.*	1 or more doses				

*Covered by the Vaccine Injury Compensation Program

☐ For all persons in this category who meet the age requirements and who lack evidence of immunity (e.g. lack documentation of vaccination or have no evidence of prior infection)

■ Recommended if some other risk factor is present (e.g., based on medical, occupational, lifestyle, or other indications)

☐ No recommendation

FIGURE 3.3
Recommended adult immunization schedule, by vaccine and age group—United States, 2010. From the Centers for Disease Control and Prevention. Recommended adult immunization schedule—United States, 2010. *MMWR* 2010;59(1).

Two vaccine-preventable diseases that occur commonly in the elderly with great risk for morbidity and mortality are influenza and viral pneumonia. Influenza results in approximately 42.7 million hospitalizations and deaths annually. Despite this high number and the availability of a preventable vaccine, less than 60% of community-dwelling older adults get vaccinated each year.

A major Healthy People 2010 objective is to increase influenza vaccination among all older adults, especially those with the following:

■ Respiratory disorders

■ Chronic heart diseases

■ Chronic renal disease, and

■ Immunosuppression

Vaccination is contraindicated in people in those who have experienced a reaction to the vaccine in the past. Pneumonia is an infectious disease caused by several possible organisms.

■ Pneumonia is the leading cause of death from infectious disease in the United States.

■ It is the sixth leading cause of death overall.

■ Estimates indicate that pneumococcal infections are responsible for approximately 100,000 deaths per year.

■ Pneumonia vaccination is recommended every 10 years or more frequently in high-risk populations.

■ Many older adults are unvaccinated against pneumonia.

■ Pneumonia vaccine is effective at preventing 56% to 81% of viral infections.

■ Pneumonia vaccine is estimated to prevent 80% of pneumonia-related deaths.

■ The vaccine is not useful in some immunocompromised patients.

Indications for the pneumonia vaccine:

■ Everyone older than 65 years

■ People aged 2 to 64 years who have chronic illness or live in high-risk areas

■ Older adults with chronic lung, heart, kidney, sickle cell disease, or diabetes.

SECONDARY PREVENTION (SCREENING)

Secondary prevention refers to methods and procedures to detect the presence of disease in the early stages so that effective treatment and cure are more likely. Routine mammograms, hypertension screening, and prostate-specific antigen (PSA) blood tests are a few examples of this type of screening.

Strategies for detecting disease at an early stage involve annual physical examinations; laboratory blood tests for tumor markers, cholesterol, and other highly treatable illnesses; and diagnostic imaging for the presence of internal disease. Secondary disease-specific early detection guidelines are discussed in the following sections.

CARDIOVASCULAR DISEASE PREVENTION

Secondary prevention efforts to detect early signs and symptoms of cardiovascular disease focus on screening for the risk factors of hypertension (HTN) and cholesterol levels to reduce the morbidity and mortality rates associated with diseases such as coronary heart disease (CHD) and the occurrence of myocardial infarction (MI) and stroke.

The U.S. Preventive Services Task Force (USPSTF) recommends screening at least every 2 years for adults, with more frequent screening if the blood pressure readings are borderline. Blood pressure management should follow the guidelines of the JNC-VII criteria for assessment and management blood pressure, which are listed in Table 3.1. Management guidelines will be discussed in greater detail in Chapter 5.

TABLE 3.1

American Heart Association Cholesterol Guidelines

Total Cholesterol Level	Category
Less than 200 mg/dL	Desirable level that puts you at lower risk for coronary heart disease. A cholesterol level of 200 mg/dL or higher raises your risk.
200–239 mg/dL	Borderline high
240 mg/dL and above	High blood cholesterol. A person with this level has more than twice the risk of coronary heart disease as someone whose cholesterol is below 200 mg/dL.
HDL Cholesterol Level	**Category**
Less than 40 mg/dL (for men) Less than 50 mg/dL (for women)	Low HDL cholesterol. A major risk factor for heart disease.
60 mg/dL and above	High HDL cholesterol. An HDL of 60 mg/dL and above is considered protective against heart disease.
LDL Cholesterol Level	**Category**
Less than 100 mg/dL	Optimal
100–129 mg/dL	Near or above optimal
130–159 mg/dL	Borderline high
160–189 mg/dL	High
190 mg/dL and above	Very high
Triglyceride Level	Category
Less than 150 mg/dL	Normal
150–199 mg/dL	Borderline high
200–499 mg/dL	High
500 mg/dL and above	Very high

From the American Heart Association, *http://www.americanheart.org/presenter .jhtml?identifier=4500*

USPSTF states that there is insufficient evidence to recommend for or against routine screening asymptomatic older adults for cholesterol. However, given the lack of evidence, individual decisions to screen this population must be made between the patient and their health care provider. AHA normal ranges for cholesterol are listed in Table 3.1.

First line treatment for elevated cholesterol levels are therapeutic life-style changes including diet and exercise. Treatment with medications is

TABLE 3.2

American Diabetes Association Ranges for Fasting Blood Glucose

Glucose Level	Indication
From 70 to 99 mg/dL	Normal fasting glucose
From 100 to 125 mg/Dl	Impaired fasting glucose (prediabetes)
126 mg/dL and above on more than one testing occasion	Diabetes

the next line of therapeutic management. Management guidelines for the treatment of specific lipid values are discussed in greater detail in Chapter 5.

DIABETES

Type II diabetes is a substantial problem among older adults. Estimates have indicated that up to 20% of the U.S. population will have developed type II DM by the age of 75 years. The American Diabetes Association recommends screening for type II diabetes in older adults every 3 years with a fasting plasma glucose test. Interpretation of fasting blood sugar levels are listed in Table 3.2. The American Diabetes Association now also recommends that a Hemoglobin A1C test is also diagnostic of diabetes with levels of HgA1C between 5.7% to 6.4% indicating prediabetes and an A1C level of 6.5% or higher being diagnostic of diabetes.

CANCER

Approximately 75% of all cancers occur among older adults, which at present constitute only about 13% of the population. Individuals aged 65 and older were found to account for 56% of all cases of breast cancer and 80% of all prostate cancer cases in 2002. Clearly, advanced age is a risk factor for the development of cancer. But, older adults are also more likely to be diagnosed with cancer at an advanced stage when the cancer is less amenable to treatment and increased morbidity and mortality are more likely. Cancer diagnosis and mortality are highly associated with factors such as genetics, race, and socioeconomic status. For both older men and women, lung cancer remains the highest cause of mortality. Lung cancer is followed by prostate cancer and colorectal cancer for older men and breast cancer and colorectal cancer for older women. There are no routine screening tests for lung cancer beyond an annual physical examination and review of systems. Screening for the other leading causes of cancer among older adults remains controversial and is discussed in the following sections.

Mammography was once considered to be the most effective screening tool to detect breast cancer, along with an annual Clinical Breast Exam (CBE) for women 40 and older. USPSTF recommended both a CBE and mammography every year beginning at age 40. However, in late 2009, current evidence was synthesized resulting in a revised recommendations to screen women aged 50 to 74 every 2 years. USPSTF states that there is insufficient evidence to recommend for or against routine mammography for women over the age of 75 as well as continued teaching of self-breast examinations (SBE). It should be noted that the decision to screen every year or not should be made between the patient and their health care provider. Moreover, the American Cancer Society continues to recommend annual mammography and a CBE every 3 years in all women over the age of 40 and continuing while the woman is in good health. (Retrieved from *http://www.cancer.org/docroot/ped/content/ped_2_3x_acs_cancer_detection_guidelines_36.asp*)

Controversy exits as to whether the PSA test should be used to screen older men for the presence of prostate cancer, as the goal of screening is to decrease mortality and improve quality of life. USPSTF has recently recommended that men over 75 years of age abstain from PSA screening because of limited benefit and increased risk for physical and psychological harm. Normal PSA values are between 0 and 4.0 ng/mL; values greater than 4.0 may warrant additional follow-up dependent on a number of patient characteristics including, but not limited to, age, ethnicity, body mass index, height, and a family history of prostate cancer. PSA change over time may be a more sensitive indicator of prostate activity rather than a static PSA value. Elevated PSA levels may also be the result of benign prostatic hypertrophy, older age, inflammation, or ejaculation within 2 days of testing. Values lower than 4.0 in African-American men and those who are obese also call for additional follow-up by a health care provider as research has shown that these factors may result in high risk for prostate cancer (American Cancer Society, 2008; Freedland et al., 2008). The PSA is only a screening tool for prostate cancer. Diagnosis of prostate cancer is confirmed following biopsy guided by transrectal ultrasound.

The vast majority of colon cancer cases (over 90%) are diagnosed in individuals aged 50 and older. The earlier the cancer is diagnosed, the higher the survival rate with diagnosis. The American Cancer Society recommends the following screening tests to detect colon cancer in all people beginning at the age of 50:

■ Flexible sigmoidoscopy every 5 years (followed by colonoscopy if test is positive), or

■ Colonoscopy every 10 years, or

■ Double-contrast barium enema every 5 years (followed by colonoscopy if test is positive), or

■ CT colonography (virtual colonoscopy) every 5 years (followed by colonoscopy if test is positive).

(Retrieved from *http://www.cancer.org/docroot/ped/content/ped_2_3x_acs_ cancer_detection_guidelines_36.asp*)

OSTEOPOROSIS

Osteoporosis affects one in two women and one in five men and results in approximately 230,000 fractures each year. (Retrieved from *http://www .nos.org.uk/NetCommunity/Page.aspx?pid=328&srcid=312*). Osteoporosis is a disease with a vast impact on older adults, especially post menopausal women. The disease weakens bones and places where older adults are at high risk for fracture. Risk factors for osteoporosis include (a) small, thin women who have fair skin and light hair and eyes, (b) older adults with a family history of osteoporosis, (c) postmenopausal women, (d) women over age 65, (e) men over age 80, and (f) sustained BMI more than 22. In addition, older individuals who consume a diet low in calcium, smoke, use excess alcohol or caffeine, and live a sedentary lifestyle are at higher risk for developing the disease.

Bone density testing is recommended for all women over the age of 65, postmenopausal women with major risk factors, everyone over the age of 50 with a osteoporotic fracture, all individuals taking long-term corticosteroids, men with hypogonadal conditions, men over the age of 70, and patients with disease associate bone loss or fracture (Ayoub, 2008). While multiple techniques and instruments are available to measure bone density, the most commonly used technique is DEXA (Dual Energy X-ray Absorptiometry). The results of these tests are interpreted in T- and Z-scores. A T-score refers to the number of standard deviations below the mean for a young adult with optimum bone density. The Z-score is the number of standard deviations below the mean of an average person of the same age. T- and Z-scores vary by patient ethnicity. The World Health Organization (1994) has provided the following guidelines to interpret T-scores based on bone density in men and women of all ethnic groups:

- Normal bone: T-score better than −1

- Osteopenia: T-score between −1 and −2.5

- Osteoporosis: T-score less than −2.5

The National Osteoporosis Foundation recommends treatment when a T-score of less than −2.0, or −1.5 with a major risk factor such as osteoporotic fracture, cigarette smoking, or weight less than 127 lbs. Treatment recommendations will be discussed in Chapter 5. The North American Menopause Society (2006) recommendations for prevention of osteoporosis include diets adequate in calcium and vitamin D with a total requirement 1,200 mg of Calcium and 400 to 600 IU of vitamin D each day.

TERTIARY PREVENTION (DISEASE MANAGEMENT)

While much can be done to prevent and detect disease at an early treatable stage, the average older adult has three chronic medical illnesses. With appropriate disease management, the impact of these diseases on quality and quantity of life may be minimized. Tertiary prevention strategies are needed after the disease or condition has been diagnosed and treated in an attempt to return the client to an optimum level of health and wellness despite the disease or condition. Physical, occupational, and speech pathology services following a cerebrovascular accident are typical examples of tertiary prevention strategies. These management strategies will be covered in more detail in Chapter 5.

REFERENCES

American Cancer Society. (2008). *Cancer facts & figures 2008.* Atlanta, GA: American Cancer Society. Accessed January 3, 2009, from http://www.cancer.org/acs/groups/content/@nho/documents/document/2008cafffinalsecuredpdf.pdf

Ayoub, W. T. (2008). Diagnostic tests and interpretation. In S. H. Guelder, T. N. Grabo, E. D. Newman, & D. R. Cooper (Eds.), *Osteoporosis clinical guidelines for prevention, diagnosis and management* (pp. 33–45). New York: Springer Publishing Company.

Freedland, S. J., Wen, J., Wuerstle, M., Shah, A., Lai, D., Moalej, B., et al. (2008). Obesity is a significant risk factor for prostate cancer at the time of biopsy. *Urology. 72*(5), 1102–1105.

Frighetto, L., Marra, C., Bandali, S., Wilbur, K., Naumann, T., & Jewesson, P. (2004). An assessment of quality of sleep and the use of drugs with sedating properties in hospitalized adult patients. *Health and Quality of Life Outcomes, 2*(17), 1–10.

Sarna, L., & Bialous, S. A. (2010). Using evidence based guidelines to help patients stop smoking. *American Nurse Today, 5*(1), 44–48.

The North American Menopause Society. (2006). The role of calcium in peri- and postmenopausal women: 2006 position statement of the North American Menopause Society. *Menopause, 13*(6), 862–877; quiz 878–879.

U.S. Department of Health and Human Services. (2001). *Healthy people 2010.* Washington, DC: U. S. Government Printing Office.

World Health Organization. (1994). *Assessment of fracture risk and its application to screening for postmenopausal women.* Geneva, Switzerland: World Health Organization.

TEST QUESTIONS

1. MC is a 69-year-old Caucasian female who has agreed to take a DEXA assessment to determine her bone density. In interpreting the results, you know that normal bone T-scores are one of the following:

A. T-score between −1 and −2.5

B. T-score better than −1

C. T-score less than −2.5

D. T-score above −2.5

2. There are several barriers to health promotion among olders adults. Which type of theory provides as an example that facilitates health promotion in this population?

A. Nursing grand theory

B. Sociological aging theory

C. Motivational theory

D. Eccentricity theory

3. A 68-year-old woman was seen by her cardiologist for advice in beginning an exercise program and asks you how much she should plan on exercising: Your response would be to make sure she:

A. Increases the consistency of her heart rate over time

B. Continues until she can no longer breathe regularly

C. Participates in moderately intense aerobic exercise 30 minutes a day, most days a week

D. Participates in aerobic exercise 30 minutes a day, every day of the week.

4. A 76-year-old man has recently been diagnosed with type II diabetes. He would like to begin exercising to enhance his blood sugar control and would like ideas on how to best design a program that he will stick with. What would your response be?

   A. Begin an exercise program with 30 to 60 minutes of vigorous exercise each day.

   B. Avoid drinking water when exercising.

   C. Add a family member or friend to your exercise program to increase adherence.

   D. Dizziness is common when exercising and should be ignored.

5. Primary prevention activities are designed to:

   A. Prevent disease before it occurs.

   B. Detect disease at an earlier, more treatable stage.

   C. Manage disease, so it does not get worse.

   D. Eradicate all diseases from the nation.

6. M.C., a newly admitted nursing home patient, just had her first hepatitis B vaccination. She questions you regarding when her next injection in the series should be scheduled. What is your reply?

   A. As soon as we can schedule the immunization

   B. 1 month

   C. 6 months

   D. She will need a booster in about 5 years.

7. You are providing an educational program on good nutrition to a local senior center. You explain to the population that nutrition is an example of which type of prevention?

   A. Primary

   B. Secondary

   C. Tertiary

   D. Preventative

8. In providing teaching to Ms. Carmen, a 73-year-old menopausal woman, it is important to inform her that the risk factors for osteoporosis include

   A. Obesity

   B. Active lifestyle

   C. BMI below22

   D. Diets rich in calcium

9. Mr. J is complaining about problems in sleeping. Sleep complaints among older adults commonly involve which of the following?

   A. Difficulty falling asleep

   B. Frequent nighttime sleepiness

   C. Heavy dependence on medications for sleep

   D. Noisy environments

10. Regarding the sleep patterns of older adults, nurse practitioners should know that

    A. Older adults are more tolerant to shifts in the sleep-wake cycle.

    B. Daytime napping of many older adults seems to compensate for nighttime sleep disturbances.

    C. Rapid-eye-movement sleep increases with age.

    D. Older adults have a higher quality of sleep than younger adults.

11. Mrs. Jasmine is an 84-year-old patient complaining of problems in sleeping and requests a sleep agent. Which of the following medications would be safe to give her?

    A. Ambien

    B. Benadryl

    C. Halcion

    D. Nidularium

12. Hypertension is frequently seen in geriatric clients and is correlated with other chronic illnesses. Which of the following blood pressure readings is consistent with diagnosis of stage I hypertension?

    A. 154/92

    B. 140/90

    C. 165/89

    D. 148/78

13. One of the greatest barriers to successful interventions to help problem older drinkers is that

    A. Older adults do not usually drive, so intoxication while driving is not detected.

    B. Nurses and health care professionals fail to detect problem alcohol use.

    C. Many of the medications taken by older adults mimic the effects of alcohol.

    D. Alcoholism occurs so rarely in the elderly that interventions are usually not necessary.

14. You are an NP in the emergency department. The CAGE questionnaire is helpful in this setting for assessing

    A. Readiness for smoking cessation

    B. Alcohol use

    C. Safe sex practices

    D. Amount of water drunk each day

15. As an NP in private practice, you are reviewing the results of a 67-year-old patient's colonoscopy. The results show no family history, risk factors, or abnormal findings and the patient asks when he will need another colonoscopy. What would your reply be?

    A. 3 years

    B. 5 years

    C. 10 years

    D. One colonoscopy over the age of 65 is sufficient.

4

Assessment of Acute and Chronic Illness

History and Physical Exam Considerations

The foundation for effective GNP plans of care is a thorough and comprehensive health assessment. The health assessment begins with a chief complaint and health history and review of systems. Physical examinations may include comprehensive head to toe examinations or could be targeted toward a specific or regional system. Laboratory and other diagnostic testing are usually conducted to provide additional health assessment information. Together, the subjective and objective data acquired from the health assessment provide the information for a plan for care. Among older adults, the traditional health assessment guidelines and standards are followed, with very few variations for the older adult population. This chapter reviews the elements of a comprehensive health assessment for an older adult, with some special considerations for this population.

HEALTH HISTORY

The health assessment always begins with a health history. This is usually the first meeting between the older adult and the GNP, and it marks the beginning of the therapeutic relationship. GNPs should focus on gaining the trust of older adult clients. A sufficient amount of time should be set aside for the health history so that the older adult does not feel rushed. Normal changes of aging result in an overall slowing down of response time. Older adults may have difficulty extracting dates and details from memory. There are many other challenges to getting a good healthy history from older adults, including the following:

- Age (older adults have a longer story to tell)

- Memory

- Tendency to underreport

- Communication difficulties (hearing impairments, language differences, and aphasias)

It is important to allow older adults time to think about their health history so as not to cause frustration about an inability to provide details surrounding former medical and surgical events. Older adults may withhold certain medical information from the interviewer because:

- The information may be too distressing to discuss.

- The client may fear the consequences of their health problems. Memories of painful tests or the fear of a stressful diagnosis may cause the older adult to minimize symptoms.

- The client may fear being a burden on the health care system or on their children and thus hide or minimize symptoms of disease.

A health history includes the following:

- Past medical history

- Past surgical history

- Cultural background

- Sources of social support

- Sources of financial support

- Occupation/retirement status

- Education

- Living arrangements

- Health promotion behaviors

  - Smoking

  - Alcohol use

  - Sleep patterns

  - Diet (use 24-hour recall)

  - Exercise

  - Use of herbal supplements

- Medications (including herbals and over-the-counter medications)
- Presence of common problems of aging
  - Dementia
  - Depression
  - Musculoskeletal disorders (osteoarthritis)
  - Sensory changes
  - Urinary function
  - Health literacy

A thorough review of systems includes the following:

- Cardiovascular system
- Respiratory system
- Peripheral vascular system
- Integumentary system
- Gastrointestinal system
- Genitourinary system
- Musculoskeletal system (ambulation)
- Neurological system (including senses)

It is critically important among older adults also to assess function and cognition as precipitating symptoms of illness in older adults. A sudden decline in functional status or a change in ability to independently complete activities of daily living (bathing, dressing, toileting, eating, transferring, and ambulating) often signals the onset of physiological disease among older adults. Standardized assessment instrument such as the Katz Index is an excellent functional assessment tool that has been used widely in many health care settings to assess function among older adults (see Figure 4.1).

Moreover, acute change in cognitive status may be the first presenting sign of illness among older adults. This is true for both cognitively intact and cognitively impaired older adults. Because altered cognitive status is one of the more commonly occurring symptoms of disease among older adults, cognitive assessment using a valid and reliable instrument such as the Mini-Cog is appropriate (see Exhibit 4.1).

Katz Index of Independence in Activities of Daily Living

ACTIVITIES POINTS (1 OR 0)	INDEPENDENCE: (1 POINT) NO supervision, direction or personal assistance	DEPENDENCE: (0 POINTS) WITH supervision, direction, personal assistance or total care
BATHING Points: _____	(1 POINT) Bathes self completely or needs help in bathing only a single part of the body such as the back, genital area or disabled extremity.	(0 POINTS) Need help with bathing more than one part of the body, getting in or out of the tub or shower. Requires total bathing.
DRESSING Points: _____	(1 POINT) Gets clothes from closets and drawers and puts on clothes and outer garments complete with fasteners. May have help tying shoes.	(0 POINTS) Needs help with dressing self or needs to be completely dressed.
TOILETING Points: _____	(1 POINT) Goes to toilet, gets on and off, arranges clothes, cleans genital area without help.	(0 POINTS) Needs help transferring to the toilet, cleaning self or uses bedpan or commode.
TRANSFERRING Points: _____	(1 POINT) Moves in and out of bed or chair unassisted. Mechanical transfer aides are acceptable.	(0 POINTS) Needs help in moving from bed to chair or requires a complete transfer.
CONTINENCE Points: _____	(1 POINT) Exercises complete self control over urination and defecation.	(0 POINTS) Is partially or totally incontinent of bowel or bladder.
FEEDING Points: _____	(1 POINT) Gets food from plate into mouth without help. Preparation of food may be done by another person.	(0 POINTS) Needs partial or total help with feeding or requires parenteral feeding.

TOTAL POINTS = _____ 6 = High (*patient independent*) 0 = Low (*patient very dependent*)

Adapted from Katz S., Down, TD, Cash, HR, S. Getz ,R.O. (1970) progress in the development of the index of ADL. *Gerontologist* 10:20-30. Copyright ®. The Gerontological Society of America. Reproduced [Adapted] by permission of the publisher.

FIGURE 4.1
Katz ADL index

PHYSICAL ASSESSMENT

Following the health history and a complete review of systems, a head-to-toe physical examination should be conducted. This is how objective data are obtained to form diagnoses.

Evaluate the patient's vital signs:

- Temperature—response to infection among older adults varies greatly; some older adults respond to infections with elevated temperatures and others with aggressive infections show no febrile response. Fever may be blunted among older adults because of the following:

  - Diminished production and reduced response of pyrogens

  - Lower baseline temperature

EXHIBIT 4.1 The Mini-Cog

Administration

1. Instruct the patient to listen carefully and remember three unrelated words and then to repeat the words.

2. Instruct the patient to draw the face of a clock, either on a blank sheet of paper or on a sheet with the clock circle already drawn on the page. After the patient puts the numbers on the clock face, ask him or her to draw the hands of the clock to read a specific time.

3. Ask the patient to repeat the three previously stated words.

Scoring

Give 1 point for each recalled word after the clock-drawing test (CDT) distractor.

Patients recalling none of the three words are classified as demented (score = 0).

Patients recalling all three words are classified as nondemented (score = 3).

Patients with intermediate word recall of one or two words are classified based on the CDT (abnormal = demented; normal = nondemented).

The CDT is considered normal if all numbers are present in the correct sequence and position, and the hands readably display the requested time.

Note. From "The Mini-Cog: A Cognitive 'Vital Signs' Measure for Dementia Screening in Multi-lingual Elderly," by S. Borson, J. Scanlun, M. Brush, P. Vitallano, and A. Dokmak, 2000, *International Journal of Geriatric Psychiatry, 15*(11), pp. 1021–1027 Copyright John Wiley & Sons Limited. Reproduced with permission.

- Impaired immunity

- Impaired ability to regulate heat and cold

- Pulse between 60 and 100 beats per minute—note irregular rhythms and follow up with electrocardiogram testing if necessary.

- Respiration (12 to 18 breaths per minute)

- Measurements of height, weight, and body mass index (BMI) are essential to develop a baseline for further comparison of nutritional and hydration levels as well as bone loss. BMIs of less than 25 are considered ideal. BMI parameters are as follows:

  - Below 18.5 = underweight.

  - Between 18.5 and 24.9 = normal.

  - 25 to 29.9 = overweight.

  - 30 and above = obese.

- Blood pressure should be evaluated in the sitting, immediate standing, and 1-minute standing positions, especially if the older adult is taking antihypertensive medications. Decreases in blood pressure of more than 20 mm Hg are indicative of orthostatic hypertension and require further evaluation. Blood pressure readings should follow The Seventh Report of the Joint National Committee on Prevention, Detection, Evaluation, and Treatment of High Blood Pressure JNC-VII blood pressure guidelines (See Table 4.1).

It is helpful to keep in mind the following basic strategies for hypertension management:

- Blood pressure should be assessed and managed before it gets too high.

- In people over age 50, systolic blood pressure is important and should be managed effectively.

- Two or more antihypertensive medications are often necessary to maintain control.

- Continued evaluation is often necessary, so maintenance of the therapeutic GNP–client relationship is essential.

In addition to vital signs, the head-to-toe physical assessment includes checking the following:

- Skin

  - Hemangiomas

  - Liver spots

  - Harmless senile lentigines

  - Inflamed skin tags (skin projections)

  - Keratoses, precancerous, and cancerous lesions

  - Herpes zoster

  - Pressure ulcers

  - Dryness

- Hair growth and nails

  - Uniformity

  - Diminished hair growth

  - Fungal infections of the nails

TABLE 4.1

JNC-VII Blood Pressure Guidelines

The JNC-VII criteria for blood pressure

BP Classification	SBP mmHG		DBP mmHG
Normal	<120	AND	<80
Prehypertensive	120–139	OR	80–89
Stage I Hypertension	140–159	OR	90–99
Stage II Hypertension	≥160	OR	≥100

- Head and neck

  - Lesions or trauma.

  - Evaluation of the sclera for whiteness.

  - Notation of the arcus senilis (grayish arc surrounding the cornea and caused by lipid deposits on the cornea, not necessarily associated with high blood cholesterol).

  - Visual acuity

  - Central vision (ability to see fine details, read, and recognize faces).

  - Evaluate for cataracts and macular degeneration (the leading cause of vision loss among older adults) and refer to an ophthalmologist for follow-up of abnormal findings.

  - Identify the tympanic membrane and light reflex in the ear.

  - Palpate nose for tenderness and signs and symptoms of infection.

  - Evaluate mouth and teeth for deviations from normal and referrals made to a dentist for further management of mouth and tooth disorders.

  - Palpate thyroid gland for enlargement and nodules. There should be no change in thyroid structure or function as patients age.

- Heart and lungs

  - Evaluate the carotid arteries and jugular veins in the neck—they should be symmetrical, nonbounding, nondistended, and absent of bruits and adventitious sounds.

  - Inspect and auscultate the heart beginning at the apex. The first two heart sounds should be auscultated, and any adventitious sounds, murmurs, rhythms, and pulsations should be noted.

- Murmurs (defective heart values) may be innocent (no associated signs/symptoms) or may be associated with

  - shortness of breath (SOB)

  - enlarged neck veins

  - dyspnea, perspiration on minimal exertion

- Inspect lungs and palpate for tactile fremitus and equal expansion.

- Percuss lung fields for areas of hyperresonance or dullness.

- Assess peripheral pulses, warmth, and color in extremities.

- Musculoskeletal system

  - Assess ambulation.

  - Assess joint range of motion, tenderness, and crepitus.

  - Begin at temporomandibular joint and proceed inferiorally to the ankles and feet.

  - Evaluate each joint, bone, and muscle group for abnormalities, tenderness, bilateral equalness, strength, and range of motion.

- Abdomen

  - Check for abnormal scars, pulsations, or distention.

  - Auscultate bowel sounds in all four quadrants.

  - Palpate for tenderness and masses

  - Percuss to determine enlarged liver or spleen

- Genitourinary

  - Older women should continue to see a gynecologist or primary care provider for evaluation of breast and gynecological disorders common with aging.

  - Older men should undergo an annual examination with a urologist or primary care provider for prostate enlargement or malignancies.

- Laboratory tests

  - Proper use of laboratory tests in evaluating older adults requires both knowledge of the normal ranges for age and the GNPs' awareness of the client's health and medication history.

  - Laboratory tests commonly used in assessing older adults are provided in Table 4.2.

TABLE 4.2

Common Laboratory Tests Used to Assess Older Adults

Complete blood count (CBC); hemoglobin (Hg), hematocrit (Hct), and white blood cells (WBC).

Normal Ranges

Males	*Females*
Hg 13–18 g/dl	Hg 12–16 g/dl
Hct 45–52%	Hct 37–48%

WBC 4,300–10,800 cells/mm^3

Tests for red blood cell (Hg, Hct, ESR) function and white blood cell function (leukocytes) to determine ability of red blood cells to carry oxygen and white blood cell role in infection.

Drug assays (e.g., digoxin, dilantin, phenytoin, theophylline, and lithium).

See individual tests for reference ranges.

A collection of tests used to measure the level of certain medications within the body. Helpful in management of medication dosing.

Glucose and hemoglobin A1C (HgA1C)

Normal Ranges

Glucose (fasting) 70–105 mg/dl

HgA1C <8%

Used to evaluate blood sugar levels and effectiveness of glucose management medications on glucose function among older adults.

Iron (Fe)

Normal Ranges

Serum iron 35–165 ug/L

Plays a role in hemoglobin and red blood cell function. Low iron is diagnostic for iron-deficiency anemia.

International normalized ratio (INR)

Normal Ranges

INR 2–3

Tests bodies clotting ability. Often used to evaluate response to warfarin therapy.

Kidney function tests (BUN) and creatinine

Normal Ranges

BUN 10–20 mg/dl

Males	*Females*
Serum CR 0.6–1.2 mg/dl	Serum CR 0.5–1.1 mg/dl

(Continued)

TABLE 4.2 *(Continued)*

Commonly used to evaluate kidney function among older adults.

Liver function tests (LFTs)

See individual tests for reference ranges.

Used to evaluate normal and pathological liver functioning.

Prostate specific antigen (PSA)

Normal Ranges

PSA <4 ug/L

Used to detect early signs of pathological prostate activity, such as benign prostatic hypertrophy (BPH) or prostate cancer.

Thyroid function tests (T3, T4, TSH)

Normal Ranges

T3 75–220 ng.dl

T4 4.5–11.2 ug/dl

TSH 0.4–4.2 uU/ml

As thyroid problems are prevalent among older adults, these tests are frequently used to determine thyroid function.

Vitamin assays

See individual tests for reference ranges.

Tests for function of vitamins within the body, such as vitamin X. Vitamins play an essential role in all bodily system functions.

Normal Aging Changes

Normal changes of aging are sometimes considered inevitable and irreversible. However, there is a great deal of variability in the age-related changes that occur among older adults. Individual aging is influenced by many factors that are both preventable and reversible. It is of critical importance for GNPs to understand the normal physiological changes associated with aging. In so doing, GNPs will be capable of differentiating these changes from abnormal or pathological organ system changes. These changes are discussed in the following sections, along with necessary nursing interventions.

CARDIOVASCULAR SYSTEM

■ The heart becomes larger and occupies more space in the chest.

■ There is a reduction in the amount of functional muscle mass of the heart.

TABLE 4.3

Common Heart Sounds

	Aortic	Pulmonic	Tricuspid	Mitral
Location	2nd intercostal space at the right sternal border	2nd intercostal space at the left sternal border	4th or 5th intercostal space at the left lower sternal border	5th intercostal space near the left midclavicular line
Loudest sound	S2	S2	S1	S1

- There is a decreased amount of blood that is pumped throughout the circulatory system.

- Normal S1 and S2 sounds should be heard. However, more adventitious S4 heart sounds are evident and may indicate left ventricular dysfunction. A review of common heart sounds is shown in Table 4.3.

- Premature contractions and arrhythmias may occur.

- Blood flow is slower.

- Wounds heal slower, impacts medication, metabolism, and distribution.

- Older adults often experience lower diastolic blood pressure.

- Older adults often experience an increased pulse pressure.

- While changes may be normal, they may also be indicative of cardiomyopathy, which warrants further cardiovascular assessment.

- Provide patient teaching regarding the role of exercise ultimately to reduce strain on the heart and blood pressure (see Chapter 3 for exercise tips for older adults).

- Fatigue, SOB, and dyspnea on exertion (DOE), dizziness, chest pain, headache, sudden weight gain, and changes in cognitive function or cognition require full assessment.

- The time of onset of effectiveness may take longer when giving meds.

- Low diastolic pressure is a risk for cerebrovascular accidents or strokes.

PERIPHERAL VASCULAR SYSTEM

- Increase in the peripheral vascular resistance (blood has a hard time returning to the heart and lungs).

- Valves in the veins do not function as efficiently and may form (nonpathological) edema.

- Inform patient that age, diet, genetics, and lack of exercise can transform nonpathological to pathological (atherosclerosis and arteriosclerosis), which can result in cardiovascular disease (CVD).

- Monitor older adults' cholesterol levels and treat with lowering agents to prevent atherosclerosis and arteriosclerosis.

- Inform patients that exercise can lower cholesterol levels.

- Discuss the right medication, exercise program, and diet for the patient as a means to slow the progression of cardiac changes.

RESPIRATORY SYSTEM

- Normal breath sounds should be present among older adults and all adventitious sounds require follow-up. Normal breath sounds are summarized as follows:

  - Vesicular sounds: low, breezy soft sounds heard over the periphery of the lung fields

  - Bronchovesicular: Equal inspiration and expiration, medium quality, heard over the mainstem bronchi

  - Bronchial: Course, loud sound heard over the trachea

- Vital respiratory capacity decreases.

  - Lungs lose elasticity.

  - Loss of water and calcium in bones causes the thoracic cage to stiffen.

  - Amount of cilia lining system decreases.

- Increases in the size of trachea and bronchi increases the risk of aspiration.

  - Cough reflex decreases.

  - Auscultating sounds is difficult due to anatomical changes, difficulty taking a deep breath, or challenges in following directions among cognitively impaired older adults. Thus, it is recommended that ausculation be done on all lung fields in a quiet environment.

  - Inform patient that pollution and smoking worsens the cilia, so smoking cessation interventions might be necessary (see Chapter 3 for smoking cessation interventions).

- Implement interventions for older adults at risk for choking.

- Frequently assess respiratory function.

- Encourage regular exercise.

INTEGUMENTARY SYSTEM

- Skin becomes thinner and more fragile.

- Skin is dry and loses elasticity (wrinkles).

- Sweat glands lessen, which leads to less perspiration.

- Subcutaneous fat and muscular layers begin to diminish, which results in less padding and bruising more easily.

- Dryness is common.

- Skin tears are common.

- Fingernails and toenails become thick and brittle.

- Hair becomes gray, fine, and thin.

- Facial hair may develop on women.

- Body hair decreases on men and women.

- Senile lentigos are normal and common in the older population.

- Promote the use of sun block, and tell patients to avoid overexposure to sun.

- Avoid the use of soaps that dry the skin and use lotion after bathing.

- Protect high-risk areas such as elbows and heels with padding.

- Refer patient to a podiatrist for effective foot care.

- Help older adults maintain their personal appearance.

GASTROINTESTINAL SYSTEM

- Assess abdomen in all four quadrants for normal bowel sounds (should occur every 5 to 15 seconds).

- Inflamed gums, periodontal disease, sensitive teeth, and tooth loss are common due to lack of adequate fluoride and mouth care in younger years.

- Decreased peristalsis of esophagus, making food more difficult to swallow

- Decreased gut motility, gastric acid production, and absorption of nutrients

- Difficulty evacuating wastes (constipation)

- Assess older adult's ability to chew.

    - Refer older adult for further oral evaluation if necessary.

    - Assist older adults in making changes in their eating habits.

    - Assess nutritional health frequently.

    - Encourage older adults to drink fluids.

    - Add bulk and fiber to diet.

    - Promote exercise.

    - Enemas and laxative medications may be given in severe situations.

    - Implement bowel habit training programs when necessary.

    - In severe cases, surgery may be appropriate to enhance ingestion and digestion of nutrients.

- Fecal impaction (primary cause of fecal incontinence) caused by

    - Polypharmacy (calcium channel blockers, iron)

    - Narcotic use

    - Immobility

    - Reduced fluid intake

    - Three Ds (delirium, depression, and dementia)

- Involuntary leakage of liquid stool (fecal incontinence) caused by

    - Loss of sphincter control

    - Decreased mobility

    - Decreased sensation in anal column

- Complications of fecal incontinence

    - Stigmatization

    - Social isolation

    - Depression

    - Fall risks

    - Skin breakdown

URINARY SYSTEM

- Kidneys experience a loss of nephrons and glomeruli.

- Bladder tone and volume capacity decrease.

- Incontinence is not a normal aging change but often occurs in response to normal changes. Types of urinary incontinence include the following:

  - Stress

  - Urge

  - Overflow

  - Transient

- Risk factors for incontinence include the following:

  - Immobility

  - Impaired cognition

  - Medication

  - Constipation

  - Diabetes

  - Stroke

- Assess for urinary incontinence complications such as

  - Falls

  - Skin irritation

  - Social isolation

  - Depression

- Teach Kegel exercises when appropriate.

- Implement voiding schedules when necessary.

SEXUAL/REPRODUCTIVE SYSTEM

- There is an overall decrease in testosterone in men, and estrogen, progesterone, and androgen in women.

- Conduct sexual assessments.

- Help older adults feel comfortable when discussing sexuality.

■ Women

  ■ Follicular depletion occurs in the ovaries.

  ■ Natural breast tissue is replaced by fatty tissue.

  ■ Labia shrink.

  ■ Vaginal lubrications decrease.

  ■ Shortening and narrowing of the vagina occur.

  ■ Strength of orgasmic contraction diminishes.

  ■ Orgasmic phase is decreased.

  ■ Artificial vaginal lubricants may help to compensate for normal aging changes.

■ Men

  ■ Increased length of time may be needed for erections and ejaculation.

  ■ Inform men to increase the time between erections.

  ■ Discuss availability of oral erectile agents.

SENSORY SYSTEM

■ Vision

  ■ Visual acuity declines.

  ■ Ability of pupil to constrict in response to stimuli decreases.

  ■ Peripheral vision declines.

  ■ Presbyopia is common, resulting from a loss of elasticity in the lens of the eye and leading to a decrease in the ability of lens to refocus on near objects and light.

  ■ Lens of the eye often becomes yellow.

  ■ Arcus senilis (ring around the cornea) may appear and is normal when aging. Arcus cornealis may indicate a lipid disorder.

  ■ Make sure older adults have a baseline eye assessment early in older adulthood and follow up eye exams yearly.

■ Hearing

  ■ Amount of hard cerumen increases.

  ■ Altered hearing is common.

TABLE 4.4

Hearing Tests

Test	Sensorineural Hearing Loss	Conductive Hearing Loss
Weber Test	Sound localizes to normal ear	Sound localizes to affected ear (ear with conductive loss)
Rinne Test	Positive Rinne; air conduction more than bone conduction (both air and bone conduction are decreased equally, but the difference between them is unchanged).	Negative Rinne; bone conduction more than air conduction

- Wax removal may be necessary.
- Hearing loss is common among older adults and may be assessed in Table 4.4.
  - Sensorineural hearing loss results from a gradual loss of high-frequency sensory neurons that conduct hearing.
  - Conductive hearing loss is a mechanical loss that is caused by infection, obstruction, or other damage to the ear structures.
- Taste and smell
  - 30% of taste buds diminish.
  - Obtain a thorough history of taste and smell sensations.
  - Conduct physical examination of the nose and mouth.
  - Obtain a thorough diet history.
  - Implement diet interventions to avoid overcompensation with sweet and salty foods.

NEUROLOGICAL SYSTEM

- Total brain weight decreases.
- There is a shift in the proportion of gray matter to white matter.
- There is a loss of neurons.
- There is an increase in the number of senile plaques.
- Blood flow to the cerebrum decreases.

- Mild memory loss is common, but cognitive impairment is not a normal change of aging.

- Help older adults maintain an active body and mind.

- Encourage older adults to participate in cognitive activities.

TEST QUESTIONS

1. During his 3-month check up, J.C, a 66-year-old male patient, states that he is concerned because he notices a light-colored ring around the iris of his eye. What is the most appropriate response by the GNP?

   A. Tell J.C. that this ring indicates a potential serious medical problem and refer him to an opthamologist.

   B. Report this information to the consulting physician to make sure it is nothing serious.

   C. Explain to J.C. that this is a normal age-related change that occurs within the eye.

   D. Tell J.C. that this condition could cause complications and must be monitored closely.

2. A few weeks after admission to a rehabilitation facility following hip replacement surgery, B.V. developed sudden onset-cognitive changes. The GNP would most likely suspect one of the following:

   A. Urinary tract infection

   B. Peripheral vascular disease

   C. Malignant growth of a previously benign tumor

   D. Gynecomastia

3. In conducting a neurological assessment for a potential neurological disorder, the GNP must be sure to include

   A. Assessment of peripheral pulses

   B. The mini-cog or similar cognitive assessment

   C. Complete blood count (CBC)

   D. Otoscopic examination

4. B.B. is a healthy older adult presenting for an admission to physical examination. In conducting his integumentary system assessment, the GNP knows
that the older adult may manifest all the following skin changes, *except*

   A. Decrease and thinning of body hair

   B. Increased facial hair in women

   C. Fingernails more brittle

   D. Balding in patches

5. Mrs. B, 75-year-old, is at your clinic for a preoperative interview. The
GNP understands that the reason that this interview may take longer
than interviews with younger person is most likely because

   A. As people age, they are unable to hear and thus interviewers need to
   repeat much more of what is said.

   B. Aged people lose much of their mental capacities and require time
   to complete an interview.

   C. An aged person has a longer story to tell.

   D. An aged person is usually lonely and likes to have someone to talk to.

6. The GNP is interviewing Mr. L who has a hearing impairment; what techniques would be most beneficial in communicating with Mr. L?

   A. Request a sign language interpreter before you meet with Mr. L to
   help facilitate the communication.

   B. Speak loudly and with exaggerated facial movements when talking
   with Mr. L, because this helps with lip reading.

   C. Avoid using facial and hand gestures because most hearing impaired
   people find this degrading.

   D. Assess the method of communication Mr. L prefers.

7. When performing a functional assessment on an 82-year-old client with
a recent stroke, which of the following questions would be most important to ask?

   A. Do you wear glasses?

   B. Do you have any thyroid medication?

   C. How many times a day do you have a bowel movement?

   D. Are you able to dress yourself?

8. B.C. is a 91-year-old resident of a long-term care facility. Her urine is cloudy and foul-smelling, which is symptomatic of a UTI, and her temperature is 97.9 °F. As the GNP caring for this patient, you know that the temperature response of older adults to infection

   A. Is about the same as that of a young child

   B. Varies widely owing to less effective heat controlling mechanisms

   C. Is always lower than that of younger adults

   D. Depends on the type of thermometer used

9. The GNP is assessing an 80-year-old man and notices that his skin is wrinkled, thin, lax and dry. This finding is related to one of the following normal changes of aging:

   A. Integumentary system changes

   B. Increase in elastin and in subcutaneous fat

   C. Increase in the number of sweat and sebaceous glands

   D. Increase vascular flow to the skin

10. The GNP is performing an eye assessment of an 80-year-old client. Which of the following findings is considered abnormal?

    A. Loss of outer hair on the eyebrows due to a decrease in hair follicles

    B. The presence of arcus senilis seen around the cornea

    C. A decrease in tear production

    D. Unequal pupillary constriction in response to light

11. The GNP is reviewing lab findings on an 88-year-old patient and notes that her vitamin B12 level is low. A decrease in B12 among older adults frequently results in

    A. Aplastic anemia

    B. Pernicious anemia

    C. Folate anemia

    D. Wernicke's anemia

12. Difficulties in performing physical examinations on older adults include all the following, *except*
    A. Polypharmacy
    B. Lack of standards
    C. Presbyopia
    D. Normal aging changes

13. Mr. Harry Potter, an 84-year-old man, is visiting the clinic for an annual examination. The most important thing to include in the examination of an older patient, in comparison to other populations is
    A. CBC
    B. Total cholesterol values
    C. Vital signs
    D. Mental status assessment

14. In following up on the lab values of a 69-year-old patient, you note that the number of WBC commonly found in older adults is unchanged. However, the existing WBCs are often
    A. Less functional
    B. Hematopoietic
    C. More flexible
    D. Useless

15. The GNP is conducting an assessment on a healthy older adult and notes one of the following as an abnormal finding:
    A. Thoracic cage stiffening
    B. Decreased cough reflex
    C. Crackles at the bases of both lungs
    D. Less cilia throughout the respiratory system

5

Clinical Management
of Older Adults

This chapter deals with the most frequent health problems, geriatric syndromes, and comorbidities with older adults, and the pathophysiology management of these issues. All older adults are not frail, but some do fall into a frailty category, which can be used to predict negative events such as falls, mobility problems, hospitalization, how someone will heal from a health problem, and even respond to dying. Frailty is defined as having three of the following characteristics: weakness, weight loss, poor endurance, slowness, or inactivity (Ahmed, Mandel, & Fain, 2007). At times, older adults will have an abnormal presentation of symptoms and diseases, which may be further masked by functional decline (Hensley & Williams, 2010). It is paramount to listen to an older adult's family or friends who say, "She is not herself and I know there is something wrong" because most likely a health problem is causing the change in behavior. Some of these changes that may be evident and indicate pathology include new eating patterns, frequent falls, incontinence, or transient confusion. Most likely, older adults will be most impacted by problems with the musculoskeletal, cardiovascular, respiratory, or neurological systems. It is also evident that chronologic age is not synonymous with physiologic age, so making differential diagnoses based on age is not prudent (Capezuti, Zwicker, Mezey, & Fulmer, 2008).

The average older adult takes approximately 4.5 prescriptions and 3.5 over-the-counter drugs. The average individual in a long-term care institution takes about eight prescriptions, so it is apparent that polypharmacy may put older adults at a higher risk of adverse drug events (Burke & Laramie, 2004). Taking too many over-the-counter and prescription drugs than are clinically needed for an individual is defined as polypharmacy. With the many comorbidities that most older adults have, they frequently go to multiple specialists; so it is significant that the primary care provider manages the various treatment plans and results. The Beers criteria for potentially inappropriate medication use in older adults is a good tool to use when prescribing for older adults.

Nurse practitioners also have to provide MedGuides, which the Federal Drug Association (FDA) mandates to be given to patients for all drugs and samples dispensed from the office. A MedGuide is a handout explaining the medication and its action, dosage and route, adverse side effects, and interactions with other drugs. The rationale is to provide information about the side effects of each medication.

Using an electronic documentation record will greatly assist the nurse practitioner in maintaining patient medication records and in having an up-to-date list of each medication and rationale for use including over-the-counter drugs and vitamins. This list should be helpful for the provider and patient to review at least annually, if not at every visit. Reviewing the older adult's administration routine would also be beneficial.

The changes in aging can greatly alter the absorption, distribution, and excretion of drugs. Because of an increase in acidity of gastric secretions and delayed emptying time of the stomach, drugs can have quicker degradation times in the stomach even if they are enterically coated and absorbed in the small intestine. Because there is less lean body mass with older adults, drugs may become more bioavailable and more toxic. Also, many older adults have decreased albumin, which will also add to some drugs' increased free availability and potential for toxicity as there will be less albumin for binding and a greater amount of the drug will remain free. Older adults who have occasional alcohol will have a decrease in drug metabolism in the liver, but those older adults with chronic use of alcohol will have an increase in drug metabolism. Older adults may need to have lower dosages of drugs because of decreased creatinine clearance, which they may experience if they have renal insufficiency. Even with normal blood urea nitrogen and serum creatinine, they still may have decreased creatinine clearance, which would be less than 75 ml/min. The rule of thumb is to halve all dosages of older adults with abnormal BUN and serum creatinine, because the predicted creatinine clearance will be less than 50 ml/minute. The Cockcroft–Gault formula often used to estimate the creatinine clearance is CrCl = 140—person's age multiplied by person's weight in kilograms divided by serum creatinine and multiplied by 72, and for women the result of the above formula is multiplied by 0.85.

Cardiovascular Problems, Pathophysiology, Management

There are many cardiovascular problems that older adults are prone to experiencing such as hypertension, coronary artery disease, heart failure, cardiomyopathy, valvular dysfunction, dysrhythmias, peripheral arterial disease (PAD), and venous disease. Additionally, older adults experience lipid and triglyceride dysfunction and various cardiac complications because of diabetes mellitus, renal insufficiency, infections (such as periodontal disease), immunosuppressive disorders, chronic obstructive pulmonary disease, thromboembolic dysfunction, autoimmune disorders, inflammatory diseases, and certain medications prescribed for other comorbidities. Also environmental and genetic factors, poor eating, and exercise habits can negatively impact cardiovascular health.

Hyperlipidemia is prevalent with elevated low-density lipoprotein (LDL) and total cholesterol counts. Older people tend to have increased high-density lipoprotein (HDL) levels. This will assist in successfully managing the patient, but the number one goal is to always focus first on decreasing the LDL to less than 100. It is possible if the person has more cardiovascular risk factors, which require an even lower LDL to attempt to decrease it to 50. The U. S. Preventive Services Task Force (2010) recommends daily aspirin for women aged 55 to 79 years to prevent ischemic stroke and for men aged 45 to 79 years to prevent myocardial infarction (MI) as long as the potential benefits outweigh the potential harm from gastrointestinal hemorrhage. This is because the most common cardiovascular disease with older adults is caused by coronary atherosclerosis. Because aspirin has antiplatelet and anti-inflammatory effect, it is commonly used with older adults who have high risk for stroke or MI. The usual dose is 81 mg. The aspirin decreases the COX enzyme and therefore inhibits prostaglandin, thromboxanes, and prostacyclin production (Edmunds & Mayhew, 2009).

Antilipid drugs can cause serious muscle discomfort and also cause rhabdomyolysis because of the increased secretion of myoglobin with the muscle injury. It is controversial as to whether older adults who are older than 80 years should be taking antilipid drugs when they are on several medications because of the possible drug interactions and liver toxicity that can result from antilipid drug metabolism. It is especially important to evaluate liver transaminases (ALT and AST) at least biannually for patients on antilipid drugs. Also, it is necessary to tell patients not to take over-the-counter medications, such as Red yeast rice, which has Lovastatin (Mevacor) in it and would cause even more lowering of the lipids along with potential side effects, such as myopathy, liver, and renal dysfunction. Nurse practitioners follow the clinical guidelines, National Cholesterol Education Program (NCEP)—Adult Treatment Panel (ATP) III. *(http://www.nhlbi.nih.gov/guidelines/cholesterol/index.htm)*, for managing cholesterol levels. The NCEP–ATP recommend that older adults should be managed with intensive LDL-lowering therapy. The statins are recommended for maximum lowering of LDL, but they do increase the international normalized ratio (INR) of patients taking Coumadin (Warfarin), so the Coumadin dosage needs adjusting. Once the LDL is at goal, the plan should be to increase HDL to more than 55 and decrease triglyceride level to less than 150. Health teaching regarding healthy life style with daily exercise and low-fat/low-calorie diet is necessary to decrease weight and maximize health.

Aortic abdominal aneurysms (AAA) are common and present as pulsatile masses in the upper abdomen. They tend to be approximately 2 cms or greater in length when initially identified. If the patient is complaining of severe back or chest pain, the pain worsens when supine and improves with positioning forward or sitting up. It is necessary to do a CT scan to diagnose the size, which may be greatly enlarged such as more than 4 to 5 cms, which would put the person at risk for rupture. Most likely the individual with a life-threatening AAA will not have palpable femoral pulses or they will be thready. This is another sign of AAA.

Valvular problems are not uncommon with older adults. Generally, the systolic murmur is audible at II to IV grades with mild aortic stenosis. This valve problem is frequently seen with older adults and can be auscultated at the second right intercostals space and also radiates to the right clavicle and the right carotid artery. If the patient squats, the sound is louder than while supine or standing; and frequently with exercise, the patient will experience angina, dyspnea, or syncope. Also important to note with aortic stenosis, the S2 is often diminished. An S4, because of decreased ventricular compliance, is seen with older adults especially those with aortic stenosis. The INR is recommended to be managed between 2.0 and 3.0 seconds for older adults with valvular disorders unless other variables are present such as thromboembolic disease. Endocarditis is caused by bacteria, viruses, fungi, and parasites, which may be more possible to occur with older adults since they generally have more open heart surgery or valve prostheses, pacemakers, and automatic implantable cardioversion defibrillators (AICDs).

Acute Coronary Syndrome (ACS) STEMI and NONSTEMI—Many older adults with ischemia or coronary artery disease experience atypical symptoms such as back pain, nausea, syncope, diaphoresis, confusion, and/or weakness. They do not generally have classic chest pain nor do they have another common angina equivalent, shortness of breath. There are multiple symptoms such as malaise, fatigue, diaphoresis, nausea, back or arm aches, or just "not feeling normal" complaints that may indicate an *Acute Myocardial Infarction* or ischemia. Some will have a **NONSTEMI,** which is a partial-thickness MI without ST elevation. Others will have a **STEMI** that includes ST elevation causing a full-thickness MI. Myocardial ischemia is reflected with ST depression, myocardial injury is illustrated with flat T, and infarction is manifested ~80% of the time with a Q wave. Older adults die within 30 days post MI in ~25% of cases.

Dysrhythmias often manifest in the sixth decade. Depending on the type and severity of the dysrhythmia, the individual can have some cardiac dysfunction. Because of a decrease in sinus node cells with aging by the age of 75 years, most people have only about 10% functioning sinus node cells, which puts them at risk for sick sinus syndrome and other atrial tachycardias. Likewise, with older adults there is a loss of atrial-ventricular node and bundle of His tissue cells increasing the risk for atrial-ventricular blocks and bundle branch blocks. These conduction problems coupled with other cardiovascular changes occurring with an MI, such as decreased cardiac output, decreased contractility, and decreased ventricular compliance, can lead to cardiac dysfunction. *Atrial fibrillation* is common in older adults and will decrease the cardiac output by 25% to 33% depending on the person's cardiovascular status. Many individuals are not aware of the irregular heart rhythm, but some may complain of palpitations and signs of low cardiac output. Most patients with atrial fibrillation take Coumadin to prevent clots and should not take complementary agents such as Ginkgo biloba and garlic because they also prolong bleeding time.

Heart failure accounts for approximately 20% of all hospitalizations of adults older than 65 years. People with *systolic heart failure* benefit from beta blockers, angiotensin-converting enzyme inhibitors, and aldosterone antagonists. Most have *systolic dysfunction,* but there are older adults who have *diastolic dysfunction* and preserved left ventricular function. Many of these individuals have hypertension and ejection fractions more than 40%. *Diastolic dysfunction* is described as having hypertrophied myocardium and increased left ventricular end diastolic pressure; whereas, systolic dysfunction has dilated myocardium and generally ejection fractions are less than 40%. A diagnosis is difficult with heart failure as clinical symptoms are so similar and generally include dyspnea, fatigue, and edema. It is important to identify risk factors such as diabetes, age, and increased body mass index (BMI) to prevent heart failure. Depending on the individual's situation, a dual isotope stress test, echocardiogram, or cardiac catheterization is needed to provide the ejection fraction and left ventricular end diastolic pressure, which differentiates these two types of heart failure (Morris, Van Swol, & Udani, 2005). Treatment for *diastolic heart failure* focuses on symptom reduction, decreasing ischemia, managing BP, and heart rate goals. Another important factor to measure is the B-type natriuretic peptide (BNP), which is elevated with heart failure. Some still describe heart failure as *right sided* and *left sided.* The right sided is considered to be pulmonary heart disease because the vasoconstricted pulmonary artery causes great resistance for the right ventricle to pump blood through with right sided heart failure, which is also known as *cor pulmonale.* The pulmonary hypertension causes a chronic pressure in the right ventricle, which causes it to eventually hypertrophy. Then, there is more congestion in the system as the preload of the right side of the heart has difficulty moving through the lungs to the left side. In an older adult with right-sided heart failure, with ankle and tibial swelling, with jugular vein distention, sacral swelling, there will be a gradual decrease in cardiac output since the blood is backing up in the system and causing less blood to actually move through the cardiac circuit.

Digoxin (Lanoxin) levels need monitoring and should be maintained between 0.5 and 2.0 mg. The most frequent dosage of Digoxin is 0.25 mg/5 ml. Older adults should be monitored for confusion, renal function, electrolytes, especially potassium if the individual is also taking a diuretic. Because of serious drug interaction, Clarithromycin (Biaxin) is not recommended to be used with individuals taking Digoxin. Heart failure and hypertension medications tend to include an ACE inhibitor, diuretic, beta blocker, or calcium channel blocker. It is important to assess for signs of hypovolemia, electrolyte imbalance specifically with sodium and potassium, possibility of orthostatic hypotension, dizziness, and the increased risk of syncope. Most diuretics require a potassium supplement to be given concurrently. Calcium channel blockers such as verapamil (Calan) may cause constipation, so a laxative may be necessary.

Beta-blocker medications can cause decreased sexual arousal, inability to identify hypoglycemia, sadness, bronchospasm, and exercise intolerance. Hence, people with asthma or other chronic obstructive pulmonary disorders (COPD) should not be prescribed beta blockers as these drugs increase peripheral vascular resistance, which is already increased with aging and will worsen the COPD. Patients taking a thiazide diuretic will be at risk for gout because the diuretic will decrease uric acid excretion. Additionally, individuals with renal dysfunction, as evidenced by high BUN and creatinine, will need to be switched to a loop diuretic such as furosemide (Lasix). Antiplatelet and antithrombotic drugs cause increased bleeding times and need consistent and continuous monitoring to manage the patient's INR and PTT.

Hypertension is a common diagnosis for older adults and is managed similarly for any patient using the 7th Report of the Joint National Committee on Prevention, Detection, Evaluation, and Treatment of Blood Pressure (JNC 7) 2004 accessible at *http://www.nhlbi.nih.gov/guidelines/hypertension/phycard.pdf.* This clinical guideline illustrates the normal, prehypertension (120–139 or 80–89), stage 1 (140–159 or 90–99), and stage 2 (>160 or >100) levels with recommendations for management. Adults older than 50 years with systolic BP above 140 mmHg have more of a risk factor for cardiovascular disease than diastolic elevated BP. Many people older than 65 years have isolated systolic hypertension secondary to atherosclerosis and need management. Patients with longstanding hypertension who do not comply with the prescribed medications develop left ventricular hypertrophy (LVH), which includes the following EKG findings: left axis deviation, R wave in lead aVL more than 12 mm, R wave in lead 1 more than 15 mm,

S wave in lead V1 or V2 + R wave in lead V5 or V6 more than 35 mm, and QRS interval more than 0.09 seconds (Andreoli, Benjamin, Griggs, & Wing, 2010). The nurse practitioner would also want to assess for other end target organ disease such as renal failure as evidenced by increased BUN and creatinine, cotton candy balls in the eye on fundoscopy, and possibly an S4 heart sound. People with longstanding nontreated hypertension will display vascular changes known as AV nicking in their eye and also have LVH. To prevent these end target organ problems, it is crucial that hypertension be managed aggressively using the JNC Guidelines to maintain the highest quality of health.

Orthostatic hypotension—Often this is referred to as postural hypotension and is common in the older adult. Orthostatic hypotension is caused by decreased compensation for BP when the body and its circulation are subjected to positional changes. It is more common with older adults because of aging, sedentary lifestyle, varicosities, and autonomic nervous system dysfunction.

Peripheral Vascular Disease—Peripheral artery disease is due to longstanding atherosclerosis, especially the arteries perfusing the lower limbs. Older adults have arterial stiffening from decreased distensibility, endothelial swelling from inflammation, and decreased arterial lumen size, thus causing arteriosclerosis. It is understood that peripheral vascular disease along with musculoskeletal problems causes the most discomfort for older adults. The World Health Organization (WHO) recommends a three-step guideline to follow for pain management that would apply for these common discomforts/pain experienced by older adults: step one is using nonopioids, step two is using opioids, and step three is using adjuvant therapies. Because of serious central nervous system side effects, it is recommended not to use meperidine (Demerol), propoxyphene (Darvon), ketorolac (Toradol), and pentazocine (Talwin) with older adults. *Claudication* is defined as discomfort in the legs with activity and resolution of the pain upon resting and stopping the activity. This is because of obstruction of arterial blood flow in the iliofemoral vessels and is the most common symptom with *PAD*. *Buerger disease* is an inflammatory disease of peripheral arteries resulting in nonatherosclerotic lesions. It is most commonly diagnosed in one's twenties, so older adults with this diagnosis would have already adapted to this discomfort caused by *Buerger disease.*

Raynaud's disease involves random episodes of vasospasm in arteries perfusing the fingers and possibly the toes. One indication that it is Raynaud's is that cold is a trigger causing the numbness and tingling in the fingertips. *Raynaud's phenomenon* is secondary to other diseases/syndromes such as scleroderma, myxedema, or a part of CREST Syndrome. An older adult would most likely have acquired either of these arterial diseases before 65 years of age.

Older adults are at risk for developing *deep vein thrombosis* because of venous endothelial damage and hypercoagulable states. Venous stasis ulcers are also possible for older adults with decreased venous return because of varicosities and incompetent vein valves.

Respiratory Problems, Pathophysiology, Management

Older adults present with varying symptoms when they have some respiratory problems such as not having a fever and having normal chest x-rays but still having pneumonia (Burke & Laramie, 2004). A PA and lateral chest x-ray will be the best choice for all adults to diagnose pneumonia.

Cough can be a result of a variety of problems such as a cold, flu, bronchitis, allergies, lung tumor, asthma, or pneumonia. The cough needs to be worked up, and differentials need to be ruled out until the cause is determined. For older adults, it is especially important to be vigilant in assessing the patient as to what over-the-counter cough medicines or any drugs the person may be using. Most of these drugs are not effective and should be discontinued, and older adults especially with hypertension should not be taking any cold remedies with pseudoephedrine. Also, it is prudent not to prescribe cough medicine with Dihydrocodeine (Hydrocodone) unless the cough is intractable such as with lung cancer.

Respiratory Infections—Older adults may be less resistant to the common cold, sinus infections, and pharyngitis, which are extremely contagious especially in the winter months or in a long-term care facility. Acute bronchitis is most likely caused by a virus, but if the person has an immunocompromised system, he or she may develop bacterial bronchitis. Therefore, older adults need to be assessed and perhaps requested to return to the provider in a specified number of days for follow-up to prevent more serious lung infections in the lower respiratory tract from evolving. Health teaching regarding cessation of smoking cigarettes, cigars, pipes and chewing tobacco should be clarified for older adults. Evidence suggests that even quitting smoking as an older adult will have a positive impact on the individual's respiratory status. Many individuals think that cigars, pipes, and tobacco are not harmful.

Older adults who have hyperresonance need to be followed up, because this is an abnormal finding that may indicate alveolar tissue changes. Individuals with emphysema may have blebs, which may spontaneously burst and cause a *pneumothorax*. This condition requires a chest tube to reinflate the lung tissue. Additionally, *aspirational pneumonia* is most common with older adults who have dysphagia or decreased mental status. Decisions on which patients can have an oral diet must be carefully determined with gag reflex testing.

Chronic obstructive pulmonary disease (COPD) includes *asthma* (reactive airway disease), *emphysema*, and *chronic bronchitis,* which cause a decrease in expiratory airflow. Emphysemic patients tend to have hyperresonance on auscultation. Many older adults have one or two of these pulmonary diseases and, therefore, are more at risk for respiratory infections and pneumonia. All older adults should receive the pneumococcal vaccine to prevent pneumococcal pneumonia. Older adults with mild bronchospasm may need a Proventil MDI inhaler. Many older adults with *reactive airway disease or asthma* experience bronchospasm, mucus plugging, and bronchial mucosa swelling. Guidelines for asthma management can be accessed at *http://www .nhlbi.nih.gov/guidelines/asthma/* National Heart, Lung, & Blood Institute (2007). These guidelines list the four levels of severity of asthma, their manifestations, and management. Older adults may be on Theophylline (Theo-24) and need the therapeutic levels assessed periodically and should be within normal range of 5 to 15 µg. It is important to also stop the use of long-acting Beta-2 agonists such as Salmeterol (Serevent) and instead use a long-acting steroid inhaler (Chowdhury & Dal Pan, 2010). Some individuals with COPD may require supplemental oxygen, which will favorably increase most individuals' quality of life.

Tuberculosis (TB) is an airborne transmitted disease that is manifested by cavitations in the lung, which if not stopped will proceed to the bone, kidneys, and joints. TB is prevalent in many geographical areas of the United States, and older adults may be at greater risk for acquiring the *acid fast bacillus*, *Mycobacterium tuberculosis*. The purified protein derivative test (PPD) is still the most common screening exam used; if it is positive, it is generally repeated and, if another positive test result is found, the individual will need to have a chest x-ray. Older adults may have a negative PPD reading initially since their immunological response is weakened, so they should have a repeat test in 1 week to validate the negative response. Use the CDC Guidelines for interpreting the PPD in 48 to 72 hours post administration—if there are no risk factors, an individual must have 15 mm or larger induration at the site of administration; otherwise, the individual with any risk factor with indurations less than 15 mm should be given antituberculosis medication for 6 to 9 months. Follow the CDC guidelines available at *http://www .cdc.gov/tb/publications/PDF/1376.pdf* for appropriate guidelines for management. Some individuals will develop multidrug resistant TB and need second-line medications such as Pyrazinamide. There is another method of diagnosing TB via serum by using the in-tube system, which consists of three tubes coated with various antigens to trigger the release of T-cell gamma-interferon production. Results of this diagnostic test are generally available in 24 hours. The most definitive diagnostic test for active TB is a sputum culture for acid fast bacillus (AFB); however, it is difficult to obtain this test on most patients.

Influenza A (H1N1 also known as Swine Flu) and *seasonal influenza* vaccination is recommended for all older adults without an allergy to eggs or other ingredients in the vaccine. Inactivated vaccines can be given simultaneously in different arms, but attenuated, live vaccines are recommended to be given at different times (CDC, 2009). It is not possible for individuals receiving the inactivated vaccine to acquire the flu from the vaccine. All adults older than 49 years must receive the inactivated vaccine, so all older adults use the inactivated vaccine. To decrease the flu severity, administer the antiviral drug, Amantadine (Tamiflu) 150 mg BID for 10 days, as soon as symptoms begin (should be given within 48 hours of initial symptoms for best efficacy) and even before the test results are confirmed for high-risk older adults. It is most important to prevent viral pneumonia in these older patients. If during the history and physical exam the provider identifies that the first 48 hours has passed since the initial symptoms manifested, the Amantadine is not effective; so adequate rest and hydration is the best treatment.

Pneumonia, which is an acute infection of inflammation of alveoli, interstitial tissue and the bronchioles, is common with older adults especially those in long-term facilities and is generally caused by streptococcus pneumoniae. Some older adults in long-term care facilities may be immobilized and experience atelectasis from lack of mobility. Other symptoms common with pneumonia are dyspnea, chest pain, and cough. For individuals with COPD and other chronic disease, pneumonia is even more frequently seen and is often because of Haemophilus influenza. Klebsiella pneumonia is seen with immunocompromised people, alcoholics, and those who are institutionalized. Cigarette smokers are prone to pneumonia especially as they age and will complain of severe fatigue, myalgias, sore throat, nasal congestion, high fever, sweats and chills at night, and may feel so poorly that they will miss work. Upon examination, individuals with pneumonia will have consolidation, which will be identified with a PA and lateral chest x-ray, and/or percussion, which will elicit dullness. Most frequently, they will also have rales and rhonchi auscultated throughout their lungs but especially in the lower lobes. The most frequently seen pneumonia in primary care is the community-acquired pneumonia caused by Streptococcus pneumoniae and is often resolved with azithromycin (Z-pak). The nurse practitioner should determine if the older adult with pneumonia should be hospitalized and if the pneumonia is community-acquired, hospital-acquired, or an immunocompromising etiology such as *pneumocystis jiroveci,* which was formerly called pneumocystis carinii pneumonia that occurs with posttransplant patients and other immunosuppressed older adults.

Cancer of the respiratory tract is more common as one ages and especially if one has smoked or worked in an occupation that causes irritation to the lung parenchyma such as asbestos. There has been little improvement in lung cancer cure because it is a disease that is generally identified when the cancer is in an advanced stage. Older adults can acquire primary lung cancer or metastasized cancer from a different solid organ such as the breast. The *adenocarcinoma* is a form of non-small cell lung cancer and is the most frequent type of lung cancer. The most aggressive type of lung cancer is small cell carcinoma, and the least common is the large cell carcinoma. *Mesotheliomas* are highly correlated to individuals who have worked or had exposure to asbestos.

Older adults who are immunocompromised may have a *lung abscess* and require a chest tube to drain the purulent substance. They will require hospitalization so they can have antibiotics directly administered to the abscess site. All older adults from long-term care facilities or who have had previous hospitalizations and develop *pneumonia* or *a lung infection* will need to be screened for methicillin-resistant staphylococcus aureus (MRSA).

Pulmonary emboli are another potential complication of surgery or vascular disease, which may be more apt to occur in older age. It is necessary for comprehensive screening to be implemented with each older person with any history of clotting dysfunction, venous stasis, and with injuries to any aspect of the endothelial lining of the vascular bed.

Acute respiratory failure with older adults poses many problems regarding the ability of the individual to be weaned off a ventilator if they survive this acute incident. The idea of a living will and the use of palliative care need to be scrutinized for each individual person, because most people do not want to be ventilator dependent or have their loved one in such a situation. Careful Do Not Resuscitate (DNR) advanced directives will need to be implemented on each individual before this acute emergency occurs, if possible, so that appropriate management can be planned and a "good" death can be experienced.

Gastrointestinal Problems, Pathophysiology, Management

Older adults are more prone to diverticulitis, bowel obstruction, appendicitis, pancreatic disease, and cancer. It is especially important to maintain nutritional calories in the older adult who are hospitalized, because they are at greater risk for malnutrition. Assess for risk factors of nutritional deficiency, such as albumin less than 3.5 g/dL, lymphocyte count less than 1,500/mm³, recent weight loss, and a history of a poor diet. Because of changes in the GI system from aging, older adults who have Crohn disease, celiac disease, or ulcerative colitis may be at greater risk for malabsorption problems such as hypoalbuminemia or decreased proteins. This can be compounded when the older adult is not able to have a well balanced protein diet, has liver disease, or may have a malignancy which would increase catabolism. Additionally, if there is low protein, then more free drugs are available which would lead to toxicity especially with the following drugs: phenytoin (Dilantin), digoxin (Lanoxin), and warfarin (Coumadin), which are frequently taken by older adults. On the other end of the spectrum, if the individual is obese (Body Fat Index >30), the person may be a candidate for bariatric surgery, which, even with older adults, may be an effective option.

Many older adults self medicate with vitamins, iron supplements, laxatives, and antacids and need to be aware of the potential side effects and drug interactions. People with liver disease need to be carefully managed as their coagulation and ability to metabolize drugs may be impacted because of the liver failure.

Currently, there are many media advertisements and also on the internet marketing colon cleansing products that are purported to cleanse the body of toxins and even guarantee weight loss. The products generally contain some type of dietary fiber supplement and laxative. The directions also recommend drinking at least 10 glasses of water per day or having colonic irrigations to flush one's colon. Many older adults have some degree of heart failure and should not be drinking so much fluid, and rectal irrigations for people with bradycardia may be detrimental since they cause vagal stimulation. It is wise to warn one's patients that they should not participate in these cleansing processes. There is also lack of evidence that there is any benefit from this process.

Peptic Ulcer Disease (PUD)—There are defects in the gastric mucosa of the stomach or duodenum caused by proteolytic enzymes pepsin and gastric acid. Older adults have a greater propensity to developing ulcers or gastritis because of aging changes and also because so many of these individuals take nonsteroidal anti-inflammatory drugs (NSAIDs) for arthritis and other discomfort/pain caused by comorbidities. Cigarette smoking also causes an increase in acid production. All individuals should take these drugs prudently and always with food to decrease the risk of developing ulcers. Also with older adults with gastric mucosal damage, there is a lack of intrinsic factor being secreted from the parietal cells which may impact the individual's B12 absorption. Often older adults have B12 deficiency, which can cause a megaloblastic anemia that would require B12 supplementation.

H2 blockers are commonly taken by older adults especially if they take NSAIDs or aspirin on a daily basis to decrease hydrochloric acid and prevent ulcerative disease in the gastrointestinal mucosa. Many older adults have PUD caused by *Helicobacter pylori* (*H. Pylori*). There are several risk factors for *H. pylori* including lower socioeconomic status, crowded living conditions, and poor sanitary conditions. *H. pylori* will need adequate antibiotic therapy and proton pump inhibitors (PPIs) to alleviate the bacteria from the GI mucosa. With older adults, it is often the focus to treat the symptoms rather than to completely eradicate the *H. pylori*, because the side effects of the antibiotics used for eradication of *H. pylori* may not be tolerated by many older adults. There is controversy whether the H2 blockers are effective in preventing ulcerations in the GI mucosa; hence, many patients are put on PPIs. These drugs are also taken to treat individuals experiencing GERD or peptic ulcers. These patients need to be followed and have their PPI's dose and frequency titrated.

Gastroesophageal Reflux Disease (GERD)—Many older adults experience indigestion and reflux of undigested food and, in fact, may also have an esophageal injury secondary to this irritating reflux of stomach contents. Most common symptoms include edema and mucosal erosion of the esophagus. They can also have increased symptoms after eating meals if they lie down to rest or eat snacks before going to bed or have coffee, fried foods, or food with garlic. GERD is because of decreased lower esophageal sphincter (LES) tone, which enables the reflux of undigested food. Any condition that causes increased abdominal pressure can impact GERD. The Bernstein test measures the LES competence. Drugs such as theophylline, calcium channel blockers, estrogen, and nicotine can trigger these events. The treatment is generally to avoid triggers and manage initially with antacids, progressing to H2 blockers [cimetidine (Tagamet), famotidine (Pepcid), nizatidine (Axid), and ranitidine (Zantac)] and then proceeding to PPIs [esomeprazole (Nexium), lansoprazole (Prevacid), omeprazole (Prilosec), pantoprazole (Protonix), and rabeprazole (Aciphex)]. Some older adults also do well by taking a prokinetic agent such as metoclopramide (Reglan). Patients with GERD should have an endoscopy every 3 to 5 years to removal of *Barrett's esophagus*, which is when the normal squamous mucosa is replaced by intestinal columnar mucosa caused by the GERD.

Intestinal Obstruction and Ileus—Older adults recovering from surgery may develop an ileus or a neoplasm or inflammatory process, which could cause a bowel obstruction. Generally, the symptoms of this obstruction would be colicky discomfort, distention, and vomiting.

Gastrointestinal Bleeding—If the patient has severe PUD or gastritis, there may be some upper GI bleeding from the esophagus, stomach, or duodenum. This needs a gastroenterologist referral for an endoscopy. Rectal bleeding is because of a bleed from the ligament of Treitz or below and is most likely because of bleeding from the jejunum, ileum, colon, or rectum.

Dysphagia—Some older adults will experience difficulty swallowing or dysphagia, which may be caused by a mechanical obstruction or functional obstruction and seems to be an insidious problem that worsens over time. Some older adults may have denervation of esophageal muscle and relaxation of the lower esophageal sphincter which is *achalasia*. These individuals need to be referred to a gastroenterologist.

Gastroenteritis—Older adults are more prone to viruses such as gastroenteritis, which cause distended abdomen, possibly some abdominal discomfort, nausea, vomiting, and diarrhea. There may or may not be a fever. They need to be aware of the importance of proper fluid hydration and taking their prescribed medications as instructed. The BART diet (B = Banana, R = Rice, A = Applesauce, and T = Tea diet) should be explained fully to the person and followed until nausea and vomiting stop. Sugar-free Gatorade or some other sugarless mineral/vitamin drinks should be used to provide both fluid and electrolyte balance; otherwise, the individual may need intravenous (IV) hydration. It is important to realize that diarrhea and vomiting are more serious with older adults especially those with other comorbidities.

Hemorrhoids—Some older adults may experience internal hemorrhoids or external hemorrhoids, which can occur from prolonged sitting, constipation, obesity and can result in rectal bleeding. Commonly the symptoms include itching and discomfort when having a bowel movement. The recommended treatment is to provide fluids at least 8 oz/24 hours, unless otherwise restricted by a health care provider, fiber in the diet, 20 minutes of exercise every day, and weight control. If necessary, a low-dose steroidal cream applied to the anus, astringents, and/or sitz baths are recommended.

Cholecystitis—This is an acute inflammation of gall bladder generally because of gallstones, which manifest as RUQ or epigastric pain, fever, vomiting (vomiting may afford relief temporarily), and possibly jaundice. Palpation of RUQ causing inability to take a breath is called Murphy's sign. Increased white blood cell (WBC) count, liver enzymes, gamma glutamyl transferase (GGT), and alkaline phosphatase (ALP) are good benchmarks with hepatic and gall bladder damage. When managing patients with hepatic and gall bladder dysfunction it is recommended to monitor for increased WBC, increased liver enzymes, increased alkaline phosphatase, and increased gamma glutamyl transferase.

Pancreatitis—Older adults may develop pancreatic insufficiency, common bile duct obstruction, infection, or cancer which could cause pancreatitis. Common symptoms of pancreatitis are fatty stools or steatorrhea, weight loss, and severe to mild pain depending on the extent of the inflammation. With acute pancreatitis, the pain is very severe and tends to be epigastric with radiation to the back. Chronic pancreatitis tends to be because of chronic alcohol abuse.

Liver disease is caused by *cirrhosis* and a variety of infectious processes such as *hepatitis*. There is a two-series immunization vaccine for prevention of hepatitis A available. This form of hepatitis is prevalent when there is poor hygiene and water purification. The person with *hepatitis A* is very contagious and excretes hepatitis A via feces. The majority of older adults have been immunized against hepatitis B and will manifest a hepatitis B surface antibody (HbsAb), which indicates immunity to hepatitis B. If someone is not immunized, he or she should be counseled to obtain the three hepatitis B vaccines. If a person acquires *hepatitis B* who is not immunized, he or she should be given immunoglobulin and begin the hepatitis B vaccinations. To be diagnosed with positive hepatitis B, the individual will have a positive hepatitis B surface antigen (HbsAg). It may be necessary to diagnose a person with hepatitis B by testing for IgM antibody to hepatitis B core antigen if the HbsAb is negative and the individual still demonstrates the symptoms. Some older adults do have chronic *hepatitis C* because they might have had a blood transfusion over 20 years ago when the screening was not as effective. To diagnose hepatitis C, one needs to have a positive HCV RNA. With liver disease, it is necessary to monitor aspartate aminotransferase (AST) (0–31 U/L) and alanine aminotransferase (ALT) (0–31 U/L), which are categorized as transaminases. Some older adults take antilipid drugs, which can cause inflammatory liver disease, so the liver profile needs to be assessed at least twice a year to R/O liver disease secondary to the antilipid drugs. With extreme liver failure, there will be portal hypertension which is because of high BP in the portal venous system. This will gradually increase and cause more problems such as ascites, splenomegaly, encephalopathy, and esophageal and gastric varices. Eventually, the patient will have jaundice because of a decreased excretion of bilirubin. Conjugated or direct bilirubin (0.1–0.3 mg/dL) and total bilirubin (0.2–1.0 mg/dL) will increase. The unconjugated or indirect bilirubin can be calculated by subtracting the direct from the total. Advanced liver disease leads to renal failure and eventually to multisystem organ failure. *Nonalcoholic steatohepatitis (NASH)* is one type of fatty liver disease that has inflammation and liver damage, which will gradually progress to cirrhosis. The other fatty liver disease is *nonalcoholic fatty liver disease (NAFLD),* and this has fat in the liver but no damage to liver. Both of these conditions are more apt to occur with obesity. People with NASH generally have no symptoms for 20 years and then develop cirrhosis later in life.

Diverticulitis—This is a condition that is more frequently experienced by older adults and is because of an inflammation of a diverticula or diverticuli. Symptoms include left-sided abdominal discomfort, increased flatulence, and patterns of diarrhea and constipation. The individual may also have a fever. If there are positive peritoneal signs, the patient needs a CT scan. The treatment generally requires antibiotics [metronidazole (Flagyl), ciprofloxacin (Cipro), and/or bactrim (Sulfamethoxazole–Trimethoprim)], and in some cases, intravenous fluids and surgery if allowed to become a bowel obstruction. Generally, it is advised for people with diverticuli to avoid residue in their diet but increase the fiber.

Diarrhea needs to be assessed carefully and worked up to determine the cause. It can result from diet, certain drugs such as antibiotics, or from a gastrointestinal virus. There are three specific types of diarrhea. Osmotic diarrhea is due to a deficiency of enzymes to absorb sugars such as lactose. Secretory diarrhea is due to the intestine having some type of toxin, which causes water and salt to be released such as with infections. Motility diarrhea is caused by a rapid transport such as that from some antibiotics or in hyperthyroidism. The work-up of diarrhea should include three specimens to be tested for guaiac, fecal leukocytes, culture and sensitivity, and ova and parasites. If it is long term, then *Clostridium difficile* should be ruled out. It is essential that the older adult with excessive diarrhea also be monitored for adequate fluid and electrolyte balance.

Constipation is a frequent disorder experienced by many older adults and is defined as having fewer than three stools per week. A complete work-up is needed to rule out other disorders, so a rectal exam to assess for rectal mucosal disease and laboratory works including thyroid profile, complete blood count with differential, and a chemistry profile are indicated. It may be necessary depending on the results to refer to a gastroenterologist. There are also multiple drugs, which can cause constipation such as opiates, Antiparkinsonian drugs, calcium channel blockers, diuretics, iron supplements, antacids, and NSAIDs. Treatment includes good hydration and a well balanced diet with Miralax, fiber with psyllium, methylcellulose, or polycarbophil. It is important for the patients to expect some degree of abdominal bloating and increased flatulence for the first few weeks after beginning fiber.

Colon Cancer—Most colorectal cancer is believed to arise from benign adenomas or polyps, which can be identified and removed in a colonoscopy procedure. Older adults are more prone to this type of cancer and need to be screened regularly as most of these growths have no symptoms. It is important to monitor for occult blood in the stools at least annually and for patients to be aware of the importance of seeing their provider if they have any rectal bleeding.

Hematological Problems, Pathophysiology, Management

Older adults have multiple comorbidities and may have anemia, which is secondary to one of these conditions or another complication of one of the diseases. A comprehensive work-up will need to be performed to determine the etiology of the anemia.

Anemias–Generally, older adults will have anemias secondary to another pathological process such as with chronic renal disease when they may have decreased hemoglobin due to the decrease in erythropoietin being made to trigger red blood cell formation. There are a variety of other reasons an older adult may be anemic, such as impaired erythrocyte production, chronic or acute blood loss, hemolysis of red blood cells, or a combination of any of these issues. Often times, drugs may cause anemias such as chemotherapeutic agents for cancer. Also the individual may have a decrease in B12 due to a gastric mucosa ulceration, which would decrease excretion of intrinsic factor from the parietal cells and cause a decreased absorption of B12. It is important to review the patient's RBC indices, which are listed below to determine the correct management of the type of anemia.

RBC Indices

MCV = Mean corpuscular volume = Cell Size

Normocytic = 80 – 100 fL

Microcytic = < 80 fL

Macrocytic = > 100 fL

MCHC = Mean Corpuscular Hemoglobin Concentration = Color

Normochromic = 31 – 35 g/dL

Hypochromic < 31 g.dL

Hyperchromic = > 35 g/dL

MCH = Mean cell hemoglobin = Mass of the RBC

27 to 34 pg/cell = Normal

Generally, there are no symptoms unless the hemoglobin is below 10 g/dL, but the classic manifestations include weakness, fatigue, shortness of breath, and pallor. A murmur over the aortic or mitral valve may be audible along with tachycardia. A frequent anemia with the older adult is *macrocytic–normochromic anemia* which is when there is a large cell (macrocytic) and a normal color (normochromic). By viewing the MCV and MCHC laboratory data, one can diagnose *B12 deficiency anemia*, which is also known as *pernicious anemia*. Symptoms include change in mental status, anorexia, beefy red tongue, icterus, splenomegaly, and slight abdominal discomfort. Due to the slow, insidious onset of this anemia, it often goes unrecognized with older adults. Treatment is supplementation with B12. The other macrocytic–normochromic anemia is *folate deficiency*, which produces similar manifestations as B12 deficiency, but there is no neurological change. Supplementation with folate will correct this anemia.

Older adults with rheumatoid arthritis (RA), AIDS, systemic lupus erythematosus, renal failure, hepatitis, and some malignancies will also have a *normochromic–normocytic anemia* of chronic inflammation where their RBC color and cell size will be normal but their hemoglobin will be low. There are *myeloproliferative RBC disorders* that tend to occur with older adults. Some examples include *polycythemia* secondary to dehydration, overproduction of RBCs due to malignancy, and increased RBCs due to hypoxia with chronic bronchitis. Some older adults may be given Erythropoietin (Epogen) to stimulate their RBC production; however, there are multiple side effects such as hypertension and nephrotoxicity with this medication, so use of it is controversial.

Leukocyte Dysfunction–Leukopenia or a decrease in the quality and quantity of leukocytes and *leukocytosis,* which is an increased number of leukocytes, can occur with older adults as a manifestation of some pathological process such as cancer. Certainly with leukopenia, the decreased number of WBCs puts the patient at a high risk for infection. Some individuals are given a colony stimulating factor to trigger new WBC growth. It is important to order a complete blood cell count (CBC) with differential to obtain the laboratory data corresponding to all aspects of neutrophils, eosinophils, basophils, monocytes, lymphocytes, and a platelet count.

Leukemias are malignant disorders of the blood that initially manifest with an uncontrolled proliferation of leukocytes. Older adults are most likely to be diagnosed with either *Chronic Myeloid Leukemia (CML)* or *Chronic Lymphocytic Leukemia (CLL)*, which are slow to progress generally. In fact, it is common that an individual will be diagnosed with one of these leukemias and not have any symptoms if he or she is in the early stages of the disease. CML has a high correlation with people who have the chromosomal translocation, the Philadelphia chromosome. There are two major types of lymphoma, and of the two, *Hodgkin lymphoma* and *Non–Hodgkin lymphoma,* older adults are more likely to acquire Non–Hodgkin lymphoma which is associated with chromosomal translocations, infections, autoimmune diseases, and immunological dysfunctions. *Multiple myeloma* or *lymphoplasmacytic lymphoma* is also more often seen with older adults and is a malignancy of the plasma cells. With this cancer, the body produces an extremely high number of one class of immunoglobulins, which increase the breakdown of bone.

Thrombocytopenia is defined as a platelet count less than $100,000/mm^3$ and is generally caused by autoimmune disease and infections that progress to sepsis and also as a complication of chemotherapy for malignancy. Coagulation alterations can occur with older adults and can be a result of malignancy or an adverse event caused by a medication or liver failure.

Thromboembolic disease in the arteries and veins are possible, and perhaps the older adult is at a higher risk for clotting problems because of cardiovascular disease and aging.

Musculoskeletal Problems, Pathophysiology, Management—Older adults who are hospitalized and bedridden are at high risk for the problems of immobility and also malnutrition. They potentially will lose more muscle through the fast paced catabolism and gluconeogenesis of fasting if they are not being nutritionally well managed.

The United States Food & Drug Administration has put a boxed warning to strengthen the fact that taking a fluoroquinolone drug for an infectious process may increase the chance of experiencing tendinitis or tendon rupture. Although a rare occurrence (happens between 0.14 and 0.4%), an older adult is more prone to this complication especially if he or she takes a corticosteroid or NSAIDs concurrently (FDA, 2008).

Osteoporosis is a disease for all ages and involves men as well as women and especially impacts individuals above 50 years of age. Older women are deemed more prone to developing *osteopenia* and *osteoporosis*. However, there are also multiple conditions listed in the next section that further increase the possibility of older men having a lower bone density.

Secondary Etiologies for Osteoporosis in Older Adults

Long-term Steroid Therapy

Antiseizure Therapy

Lithium

Long-term Heparin Therapy

Alcohol Induced

Cushing Syndrome

Hyperparathyroidism

Hyperthyroidism

Crohn's Disease

Ulcerative Colitis

Multiple Myeloma

Bone mineral density (BMD) is the standard measurement, and individual's BMD is compared to the average peak (mean) of a healthy young adult. A woman's BMD is interpreted by subtracting the average BMD score of a young adult population from the older adult's BMD score and then dividing by the standard deviation (SD) of the young adult population (Gueldner, Grabo, Newman, & Cooper, 2008, p. 34). The patient's deviation from the average score is assessed and expressed in SDs from the mean and also referred to as a T-score. Osteoporosis is defined as a BMD score that falls 2.5 SDs below the mean, and osteopenia is the diagnosis for scores that fall 1 to 2 SDs below the mean, and normal BMD is defined as a score within 1 SD of the mean. There is another method of interpreting BMD using a Z-score, which is used for individuals below 50 years of age and compares BMD scores related to the patient's age and gender to a similar matched population's average BMD scores. Some explain osteoporosis with regards to the body mass index (BMI) and state thinner people with a BMI less than 22 are at a higher risk for developing osteoporosis.

Many women and men on alendronate (Fosamax) stay on the drug indefinitely, and newest research supports that there is no additional benefit if taking the drug after 5 years. Using bisphosphonates for a long term is thought to possibly increase risk for femur fracture that could occur without trauma and delay healing of small fractures that occur normally. So, it is best to only continue the bisphosphonates for high-risk patients with low bone density, previous fractures, and for those on long-term corticosteroids. For older adults who experience pain from fractures due to osteoporosis, Miacalcin has been proven effective. A management plan for those stopping the medication includes checking bone density annually and administering the drug if bone density decreases.

It is significant to identify people with osteoporosis or osteopenia to decrease risk for fracture. Presently, adults older than 50 years most commonly fracture their wrists; if they are older than 60, the vertebrae are the most common fracture site, and if 70 years or older, the hip becomes the most frequent fracture site.

To prevent osteoporosis, it is necessary to maintain a daily exercise regimen and a diet high in calcium and vitamin D. Bone mass density (BMD) can be increased or at least not decreased if individuals also take pharmacological therapy such as bisphosphonates, calcitonin, parathyroid hormone, estrogen, selective estrogen receptor modulators, or calcium and vitamin D supplementation. A combination of these medications is suggested for best effect given an individual's risk factors (Gueldner et al., 2008). Older adults may need supplementary vitamin D because many do not get outside to soak up the ultraviolet rays of the sun, which will convert 7-dehydrocholesterol to vitamin D. Often, a multivitamin contains only 400 IU, and therefore supplementation of vitamin D may be necessary but should not exceed 1,000 IU/day. Also, because many older adults have decreased liver and renal function, they may develop *osteomalacia* as the metabolically active type of vitamin D needs to be metabolized in the liver and kidney. The serum 25(OH) D level, which is the precursor to vitamin D optimal levels, are believed to be more than 75 ng/ml and is the benchmark diagnostic screening test for vitamin D levels. Deficiency is less than 20 ng/ml, and insufficiency is between 20 and 30 ng/ml (Mayhew, 2009). The Institute of Medicine recommends older adults above 71 years should have at least 600 IU/day; however, there is controversy on daily intake and some recommend ~800 to 2,000 IU/day (Cherniak, Levis, & Troin, 2008; Ryan, 2007).

Low Back Pain—As with anyone, low back pain with older adults can be excruciating. It is significant to be able to identify the cause, so planned interventions can be made with the patient. Negative straight leg raises bilaterally indicate that the patient is able to flex his hip 90 degrees without causing lower back pain. A thorough assessment of the patient is necessary to ascertain the cause of the pain. Discomforts from disc problems are often exacerbated if the patient is asked to bend forward; whereas, spinal stenosis has an aching pain that is relieved by sitting and worsened with arching backward. *Radiculopathy* is usually the cause of low back pain, and when the patient coughs, there is an increase in back pain. Patrick's Test is used to determine if the pain is radiculopathy: have the patient place his ankle down on the contralateral knee and then the examiner presses down on the flexed knee of the leg which has the ankle placed on the opposite knee. If pain increases in the lower spine, it is due most likely to a vertebral compression fracture. If pain is felt in the hip, then articular disease of the hip is the etiology. Or, if pain is felt radiating from the lower back down the leg, then it is most likely a radiculopathy (Williams, 2008).

Many older adults take NSAIDs for their musculoskeletal discomfort and need to be reminded to take these drugs with food to prevent complications such as gastrointestinal mucosal bleeding, gastritis, and peptic ulcer disease. It is suggested that no NSAID be recommended to older adults without writing down the dose, time interval, and that it needs to be consistently taken with food. For many older adults, NSAIDs will require the person be also placed on a H2 blocker to prevent gastrointestinal problems such as upper GI bleeding. It is thought that NSAIDs may also cause renal vasodilation because of prostaglandins, which in turn cause fluid retention and renal injury. This could ultimately cause worsening of hypertension or trigger heart failure with patients with cardiovascular disease. Taking medications on a scheduled basis will maintain effective pain management than just waiting for the pain to become excruciating and taking the medication once the pain is acute. The provider needs to reinforce this scheduling of medications with the patient and family to enhance pain control and decrease restlessness and anxiety. If the individual has a change in pain, the provider needs to assess the patient and not just send in a different pain medication prescription.

Hip pain after falling is common with older adults. If the affected leg is shortened and externally rotated, an intertrochanteric fracture is suspected; whereas, if the leg is externally rotated but the leg is not shortened, then it is probably a fractured femoral shaft.

Osteoarthritis is a degenerative joint disease that is often experienced by older adults and attributed to wear and tear. There is no synovial membrane inflammation as there is with RA, although there are synovial cysts. Generally, people experience pain, joint swelling, stiffness, and limited motion of a joint(s), so they tend to take NSAIDs to relieve the inflammation and discomfort. There is joint space narrowing and osteophytes on radiographic studies that can assist in diagnosing osteoarthritis. Often, the individual will have bony protuberances on the distal interphalangeal joints (DIPS) called Heberden's nodes and similar protuberances on the proximal interphalangeal joints (PIP) called Bouchard's nodules. The DIP joints are rarely involved with *RA*.

Rheumatoid Arthritis—This is an autoimmune disease that is generally first experienced in the individual's 20s or 30s and that continues to progress. The pathophysiology involves inflammatory destruction in the synovial membrane of connective tissue of all joints caused by osteoclast activation and tumor necrosis factor release, which cause the joint damage. There are also systemic symptoms such as increased WBC count, fever, fatigue, and high fibrin levels. It is difficult to diagnose RA initially, because many of the serum markers are not consistent from patient to patient. It is most likely going to be diagnosed over a series of appointments as the provider is able to assess the changes in the individual's involved joints. RA sufferers experience severe morning joint stiffness that can last for more than 1 hour and tend to involve bilateral joints. Adults with RA will be on many medications from the disease modifying antirheumatic drug category (DMARD) and will require continuous monitoring. At this time, only methotrexate is able to stop the progression of the disease.

Gout—This metabolic disorder related to purine impacts either the body's control of uric acid production or the ability to excrete uric acid and causes it to rise. The elevated uric acid can cause crystallization, which can advance to gouty arthritis or tophaceous gout. This is a painful disorder but can be managed by medications that decrease inflammation and stop production of uric acid or facilitate the excretion of uric acid.

Fractures—Older adults are at risk for both complete and incomplete fractures. The broken bone can cause damage in the surrounding tissue, to the adjacent nerves, and the blood vessels perfusing the bone. For adults with normal bone density and no other factors impacting healing, it takes approximately 3 to 4 months for healing. Symptoms include swelling, discomfort to acute pain, muscle spasm, and lack of range of motion. Treatment will consist of surgery and/or traction/braces/splints depending on the patient's unique situation.

Tendonitis—This condition is common with all adults including older adults and can occur with any tendon. They may be more prone to bursitis, which is inflammation of the bursa from repeated trauma.

Bone Tumors—*Chondrosarcoma* is cancer of the cartilage and tends to occur in middle aged and older adults. *Myeloma* is plasma cell cancer and occurs most often with older adults.

Endocrine Problems, Pathophysiology, Management—Older adults are vulnerable for endocrine abnormalities given their age and also other comorbidities. For example, there is research that connects vitamin D deficiency with metabolic problems, such as hypertriglyceridemia, hyperlipidemia, hypertension, and hyperglycemia, and even with cancer and cardiovascular disease (Cherniak et al., 2008). Additionally, older adults and especially those with a family or personal history of cancer, diabetes, or cardiovascular disease should be screened for thyroid annually (Syroney & Franjesevic, 2010). *Metabolic syndrome* is also common with older adults and consists of increased abdominal tissue girth, increased BP, increased lipids and triglycerides, and insulin resistance and is often present with people who have Type 2 diabetes mellitus (T2DM). These individuals generally are on multiple medications for hypertension, elevated lipids and triglycerides, and possibly, also for insulin resistance/diabetes mellitus. People who have metabolic syndrome are at high risk for an *MI*; in fact, they are at the same risk for having an MI as if they had had a previous MI.

Diabetes Mellitus—*Type 2 diabetes mellitus* (T2DM) or prediabetes (FBS = 100–110) is most likely seen in the older population versus *Type 1 diabetes mellitus* (T1DM). This form of diabetes is a result of pancreatic beta cells being replaced with scar tissue so they are dysfunctional. Genetic predisposition, central obesity, and physical inactivity all lead to this condition. In 2007, statistics revealed that 23.1% of all people above 60 have diabetes. The newest guidelines published by the American Diabetes Association (2009) recommend the glycosylated hemoglobin (HgA1c) as the benchmark diagnostic for diabetes because it can be done without fasting and is effective in determining an individual's blood sugar level. This is a change in practice because previously the HgA1c was never used as a diagnostic benchmark parameter. The normal HgA1c is 5%. Prediabetes is defined as an HgA1c of 5.7% to 6.4%. The diagnosis of diabetes occurs when the HgA1c is above 6.5%. Additionally, the traditional laboratory tests, fasting plasma glucose, or oral glucose tolerance tests can be performed. A diabetic should maintain their HgA1c at or below 7% to prevent diabetes-related complication such as a *cerebrovascular accident, coronary artery disease,* or *PAD.* Because of normal aging, there is increased insulin resistance; and when an older adult has an acute health problem, it is common for the blood glucose to be increased. Most acutely ill individuals will require a regular insulin pump to manage the hyperglycemia. It is also not uncommon for diabetics who experience an MI to be prone to heart failure post MI. One complication of diabetes that is most painful and needs careful management is neuropathy, which causes a burning sensation often in the feet. These patients may need to be seen by a pain specialist who will try multiple pain management techniques to achieve the most effective pain control. Often tricyclic antidepressants are used in addition to analgesics to provide the most effective pain management. The goal of pain management is to assist individuals to achieve the highest level of pain-free functioning and quality of life possible.

Thyroid—Older adults have some thyroid atrophy, scarring, and an increased vulnerability to inflammation, so it is more common to see hypothyroidism than hyperthyroidism with older adults. *Hypothyroidism* is diagnosed when the TSH is more than 3.0 mlU/L and the T4 free is less than 0.7 ng/dl. Often, older adults present with depression, weight loss, change in cognition, and a general failure-to-thrive versus the more classic symptoms of hypothyroidism including bradycardia, bradypnea, fatigue, weight gain, and a general hypoactivity. Primary hypothyroidism is dysfunction of the thyroid gland, and secondary disease is caused by alteration of the pituitary TSH production. Always start low and go slow with a new medication especially a drug with a long half life, such as Synthroid (Levothyroxine), when managing a new diagnosis of hypothyroidism. *Hyperthyroidism* is diagnosed when the thyroid stimulating hormone (TSH) is less than 0.3 mlU/L and/ or the T4 free is more than 1.8 µg/dl. Primary hyperthyroidism is due to disease of the thyroid gland, and secondary hyperthyroidism is caused by dysfunction of the pituitary gland. With older adults, it is important to observe for atypical presentation such as apathy, fatigue, depression, and malaise as compared with the classic symptoms of hyperthyroidism, which include anxiety, tachycardia, tremor, and hyperactivity. Additionally, it is common to see hyperthyroidism with older adults experiencing new onset atrial fibrillation or heart failure. Use a TSH to assess if hypothyroidism or hyperthyroidism with a normal range of 0.3 to 3.0 mlU/L. Drugs such as estrogen, aspirin, amiodarone (Cordarone), and some anticonvulsants medications may falsely affect T3 and T4.

Alterations of the parathyroid glands can occur with older adults. *Hyperparathyroidism* can be a result of increase in parathormone (PTH) due to another chronic disease such as chronic renal disease or due to an excess secretion of PTH from one of the parathyroid glands. *Hypoparathyroidism* is caused by low PTH levels being secreted from the parathyroid glands or secondary to thyroid surgery if iatrogenic damage occurred to one or more of the parathyroid glands.

Adrenal glands are divided into the cortex, which is stimulated by the adrenocorticotropic hormone and releases glucocorticoid, estrogens, androgens, and mineralocorticoid hormones. The medulla secretes the catecholamines (epinephrine and norepinephrine). With older adults, there is a decreased clearance of cortisol. Disorders with excessive cortisol can lead to *Cushing's disease*, which is an increased secretion of adrenocorticotropic hormone from the pituitary or *Cushing's syndrome*, which is an excessive level of serum cortisol. An older adult could also acquire *hyperaldosteronism*, which is too much aldosterone or too little cortisol and which would indicate *Addison's disease*. Problems with the adrenal medulla tend to be hyperfunctioning caused by a *pheochromocytoma tumor*, which secretes an abundance of catecholamines causing an acutely high BP.

Older adults experiencing brain tumors or treatments for these tumors may experience changes in their antidiuretic hormone (ADH) levels. For example, postcraniotomy patients sometimes experience *diabetes insipidus (DI)*, which is an insufficiency of ADH that impacts the sodium level by elevating it and also increases the serum osmolarity. The opposite findings can occur with older adults who have a brain tumor or perhaps have some ectopic secretion of ADH, which occurs with metastasis and tumor proliferation. This condition is *Syndrome of Inappropriate Antidiuretic Hormone (SIADH)*, which causes increased ADH and decreased serum sodium and osmolarity.

Immunologic Problems, Pathophysiology, Management—Older adults especially those who reside in long-term care will most frequently have skin or urine infections or pneumonia, and this is generally due to their decreased T-cell and B-cell immune function. But it is compounded if the individual also has an indwelling catheter or other invasive line. Also significant to monitoring patients' response to an infection are the immunoglobulins. IgE increases when subjected to allergens. IgA refers mostly to mucous membranes. IgM is the primary antibody to respond to an antigen, and IgG is the major secondary response to infection. Autoimmune rheumatic diseases (ARD) include RA, which is discussed in the musculoskeletal section of this chapter. High sensitivity C-reactive protein (hs-CRP) is a trend indicator to assess a patient's response to medication. It is a general parameter that is valuable to not as long as the individual has a previous hs-CRP marker to compare the present one for change. The normal range is 1.0 to 3.0 mg/L. Older adults have decreased inflammatory response due to the chronic illnesses they have and the medications they generally take for these problems.

Giant cell arteritis is a common disorder among older adults and is often called temporal arteritis. Symptoms include headache, scalp tenderness, and sometimes visual disturbances. The treatment of choice is prednisone 60 mg/day for 2 months. It is diagnosed by increased sedimentation rate and temporal artery biopsy. The remaining CBC is within normal limits. Blindness can occur if visual problems persist and are not treated due to the inflammation of the optic nerve.

Systemic lupus erythrocytosis (SLE) is an autoimmune disorder of unknown cause, which impacts both humoral and cellular immune systems. It generally occurs with women between 20 and 50 years of age, but these individuals can live to older age if they follow their prescribed management. Symptoms include a facial malar rash, alopecia, oral ulcerations, weight loss, joint arthralgias, photosensitivity, decreased urine output, and other symptoms of chronic renal disease, headache, and fatigue. They also can have pericarditis, pleuritis, vasculitis, keratoconjunctivitis, Raynaud's phenomenon, and pancytopenia. Generally, an individual must have 4 out of 11 possible symptoms to be diagnosed with SLE. People with Lupus will need to be consistently managed for their exacerbations and generally will need antibiotics, steroids, and immunosuppressants, which will need to be monitored for potential side effects.

HIV is a viral disease caused by a retrovirus that decreases the T helper cells. It is diagnosed by testing serum with the enzyme-linked immunosorbent assay (ELISA) and the Western blot test or with an HIV oral mucus test, which generates a response in 20 minutes (Mayo Clinic, 2010). *HIV virus* is most frequently monitored by the HIV viral load test to determine if the individual is having the correct response to the medication being used. Another test to assess how a patient is progressing with HIV is the cluster determination (CD4) test, which assists the provider in determining which drugs would be best used to prevent further opportunistic infections. Once an individual reaches a CD4 level below 200, the person is diagnosed with *AIDS* and becomes extremely vulnerable for all opportunistic infections and two cancers: *non–Hodgkin's lymphoma* and *Kaposi sarcoma*. Normally, the CD4 is between 800 and 1,000 cells/mm^3. Generally, once the individual's CD4 count is less than 200 and the HIV viral load is less than 75 copies, he or she has acquired AIDS. This is now considered a chronic disease and can last for years with the protease inhibitors that target viral protease and highly active antiretroviral therapy that work on reverse transcriptase. The most frequent symptoms of early positive HIV include pharyngitis, fatigue, and a fever, and as the disease progresses, the provider will be managing and trying to prevent symptoms of infections.

Sjogren's syndrome is an autoimmune disorder of the exocrine glands, specifically the lacrimal and salivary glands. Therefore, the main symptoms include dry eyes and mouth and many patients also suffer from *Raynaud's phenomenon*. However, Sjogren's syndrome is also linked with RA, lymphoma, and other autoimmune diseases, so consistent assessment and management of Sjogren's patients is needed. The general treatment includes antimalarial drugs, immunosuppressants, NSAIDs, and steroids, along with treatment for dry eyes and mouth.

Systemic vasculitis can be divided into small, medium, and large vessel vasculitis that are chronic disorders of the vessels caused by endothelial inflammation and injury. This gradually leads to ischemia and thrombosis, which can cause severe organ disease depending on which vessels are involved. *Wegener granulomatosis* affects small vessels, *polyarteritis nodosa* impacts medium vasculature, and *temporal arteritis* is an example of large vessel vasculitis. Immunosuppressive therapy and steroids are the main interventions.

Fibromyalgia is a widespread discomfort and tenderness felt on specific body pressure points combined with some of the following problems: sleep problems, irritable bowel disease, headache, mood disorders, and fatigue. There is no known cause.

Neurologic Problems, Pathophysiology, Management—Older adults are at risk for multiple changes in their neurologic system ranging from the level of consciousness and papillary changes, movement disorders to changes in cognitive status. Additionally, they may be taking medications for non-neurological problems that impact a medley of other body systems. It is important to avoid any anticholinergic or muscarinic drugs (antihistamines, H2 blockers, TCAs, antispasmodics, phenothiazines, and narcotics) with the elderly because these medications can lead to constipation, urinary retention, and also impact individuals who have *Sjogren's syndrome, glaucoma, benign prostate hyperplasia, vascular disease,* or *chronic bronchitis.* Side effects of these drugs include mental status changes, dry eyes and mouth, blurred vision, urinary retention, and drying of bronchial secretions. Delirium and dementia are discussed at the end of this section.

Migraines generally are experienced by individuals throughout their lifetime and are not a new finding as one ages. This pain is a result of inflammation and vasodilation. The headache can be very debilitating and would be enough to discourage an older adult with other comorbidities from pursuing their everyday challenges and generally would prevent them from planning a trip or maybe even volunteering on a regular basis. It is not uncommon for people with longstanding migraine headaches to experience unilateral facial numbness along with the pain and nausea. Sometimes the individual can identify triggers such as stresses, smells, or certain foods that trigger the migraine. The pharmacological intervention is similar to anyone with moderate migraines, which is to start with NSAIDs such as ibuprofen either at 200 mg/dose or 400 mg/dose. Some advocate the concurrent use of metoclopramide 5 mg (Reglan), which increases the action of the NSAIDs and manages the migraine pain effectively for many (Adelman, Adelman, Freeman, Von Seggern, & Drake, 2004). Another medication to try is acetaminophen/dichloralphenazone/isometheptene (Midrin), which is comparable to imitrex (Sumatriptan) for effective management of migraine with or without aura as long as it is taken at the beginning of the migraine (Adelman, Adelman, Freeman et al., 2004). When all else fails, it is best to use a triptan such as sumatriptan (Imitrex) or relpax (Eletriptan) that are found to be most effective with aborting severe migraines, although these drugs are most expensive and may be out of the older adult's budget for medications (Luthy, Peterson, & Wilkinson, 2008). Narcotic medications should be used only when all else fails and should be managed initially by a neurologist. Individuals experiencing *tension headaches* should be counseled to exercise, eat well-balanced meals, have an 8-hour night's sleep, and reduce their everyday stressors. Tension headaches are generally bilateral with mild to moderate discomfort but not such that it prohibits one from working or doing activities of daily living. *Cluster headaches* are more apt to occur with men and later in life. The exact etiology is unknown but is thought to be related to trigeminal nerve dysfunction. This headache presents as an everyday occurrence around the same time for a period of days and then resolves; however, recurrence is often seen. The pain is excruciating, unilateral, and generally involves lacrimal gland draining from one eye.

Transient ischemic attacks (TIAs) cause symptoms such as paralysis or paresis, garbled speech, or visual disturbances, and these symptoms must resolve within 24 hours if they are to be defined as a TIA. TIAs are warning signs for *CVAs*. Hemorrhagic versus ischemic strokes (thrombotic and embolic) occur most often in the older adult population. Most frequently, it is an ischemic stroke, and the person will need management of lipids, BP, and diabetes mellitus as well as with rehabilitation from the stroke. After a stroke, people are using hemiplegic or have some paresis and will have to engage in a rigorous physical therapy to regain their mobility.

Many older adults with a *seizure disorder* are on Phenytoin (Dilantin) and their therapeutic level should be between 10 to 20 µg/ml. Seizures that occur in old age individuals often signal a tumor or some inflammatory process and need comprehensive follow-up. Individuals who develop a seizure disorder unrelated to a brain neoplasm will need to be aware that they will have to take medications forever, not drive or work with heavy machinery, and become aware of how their body manifests symptoms that may precipitate a seizure. *Status epilepticus* is a medical emergency and is a condition that causes severe seizure activity without regaining consciousness spontaneously. Interventions for a patient with status epileticus include maintaining airway, breathing and circulation, providing a safe environment for the individual, and having the crash cart with oxygen, suction, and medications available. Often, diazepam (Valium) is given IV to break the seizure. Generally, only one-third of the causes of seizures are identified and the majority occur in the temporal lobe. Diagnostics include electroencephalogram, CT/MRI to R/O neoplasm, and a complete neurological exam. It is common post CVA to assess patients with problems processing, such as with agnosia (defect of pattern recognition), dysphasia (difficulty with communication), or aphasia (difficulty with language). Many older adults also have dysmnesia (difficulty with memory).

Due to older adults being more prone to malignancy, it is not uncommon for them to have metastasis to the brain or even a primary *brain tumor* such as a glioma. If an older adult experiences *headaches* that are more stress or tension related and did not have these problems when he or she was younger, it is considered a red flag for a thorough neurological work-up for a possible neoplastic process.

Older adults are more vulnerable for infectious processes such as *central nervous system infections* like *encephalitis*. Symptoms manifested would include fever, headache, mental status changes, seizures, nuchal rigidity, and focal neurological signs. Early diagnosis with appropriate antibiotics is a key for survival with these life-threatening bacterial and viral infections.

There are multiple *neuromuscular degenerative disorders* such as multiple sclerosis, Guillain–Barre syndrome, amyotrophic lateral sclerosis, myasthenia gravis, and the genetic disorder, Huntington's chorea, which tend to manifest symptoms earlier than 65 years of age. Each of these diseases has a separate pathophysiological process that causes the symptoms which the individual must live with and adapt. Each would be followed by a neurologist. Amyotrophic lateral sclerosis (ALS) is a neurodegenerative disease but the intellect remains intact. Currently, the only medication available for ALS patients is Rilutek (Riluzole), which is a glutamate blocker. *Multiple sclerosis* is an autoimmune disease that destroys the myelin sheath and is most frequently manifested as the relapsing-remitting type of the disease. A relapse is defined as a loss of some physical function for at least 24 hours. The other types of this neuromuscular disease include more aggressive manifestations such as primary–progressive, secondary–progressive, and progressive–relapsing.

Syncope can be caused by a variety of problems, but a diagnosis of syncope will always include loss of consciousness. Diabetes or sick sinus syndrome or a variety of other cardiovascular disorders could cause dizziness. Additionally, medications such as antihypertensives, benzodiazepines, and narcotics can cause dizziness. Dizziness that involves disequilibrium is a symptom that needs a comprehensive work-up and generally includes a testing for vertigo and *Meniere's disease*. *Vertigo* remains with the patient as long as the position the individual is in remains the same, and this is called benign positional vertigo.

Resting tremors only occur at rest and are directly related to basal ganglia disorders such as *Parkinson's disease*. This tremor is slow and generally consists of three tremors per second (Williams, 2008). Parkinson's disease is due to decreased dopamine and acetylcholine and causes degeneration of the basal ganglia, specifically in the dopaminergic pathway.

Cerebellar disease generally causes intention tremor that is more exaggerated as the hand reaches what it is targeting to pick up. The essential tremor is more likely caused by a basal ganglion disorder involving the head or trunk and is a coarse movement.

Older adults have high risk of falling and also may be involved in a *traumatic brain injury*. The injury could be caused by blunt or open force, which can result in an epidural hematoma, subdural hematoma, or intracerebral hematoma. All individuals are vulnerable for a diffuse axonal injury in the brain that tears apart the nerve fibers. This can occur as an accident or as physical abuse such as with shaking syndrome. Some older adults' injury may cause them to experience a comatose state because of the severity of their injuries.

Delirium Problems—This is a sudden process occurring over a few hours or days that causes a change in mental function along with agitation. However, it is possible to have dementia and also experience delirium. The Mini-Mental Status Tool is still used although it is controversial in terms of its reliability and validity. It is most significant that the nurse practitioner perform a comprehensive physical exam and laboratory work to rule out possible disorders and to identify others such as a deficiency of vitamin B12 or an infection that could trigger delirium and sometimes even dementia in the older adult.

Older adults are more likely to have less physiological response to infection such as a fever but present with a more serious clinical response. Often an older adult with an infection, hypoxia, or an adverse response to a drug manifests an acute state of confusion or delirium. Treatment will include management of the etiology of the problem that triggered the delirium, possibly restraints if the person is hallucinating and delusional, reorientation and reality exercises, and possibly medications to sedate the patient. It is wise to think of delirium as consisting of two problems: 1. Is the confusion and change in mental status delirium? and 2. What is causing the delirium? Delirium is caused by metabolic problems, infectious processes, and injury to neurological tissue and is considered a medical emergency. It is often due to abuse, overuse, or withdrawal of medications, so a comprehensive medication history is imperative. Sundowning or worsening of symptoms during the night is frequently seen with older adults with delirium.

Dementia Problems—Generally, the dementia or impaired cognitive function is caused by a pathological problem, and it should not be seen as a diagnosis but rather a symptom. Dementia tends to be an insidious process that can occur over months or even years but not suddenly, and its victims have no change in the level of consciousness. Older adults with Alzheimer's disease tend to be happy and fabricate stories and reminisce about happier times in their lives. The pathology of Alzheimer's is not entirely known but is thought to be caused by a decrease in the availability of acetylcholine. On autopsy, brains of people who manifested forgetfulness, short-term memory loss, disorientation, and decline in cognition and who were thought to have Alzheimer's disease had plaques, enlarged ventricles, and neurofibrillary tangles in their brains. They have good long-term memory but cannot remember the here and now and have no idea that they have lost this part of their memory. They are extremely repetitive with their stories of earlier times; whereas, people with vascular dementia know that they do not know or remember and do not fabricate stories. Generally, this dementia is linked with an earlier CVA. Their symptoms include incontinence, walking difficulty due to gait disturbance, and a flat affect. Dementia of Diffuse Lewy body disease is a combination of Parkinson's disease and Alzheimer's disease, which tends to progress quicker and develop protein aggregates which are termed Lewy bodies in the limbic system, cortex, and brainstem. These cause more fluctuations in cognitive function. The Parkinsonian symptoms include rigidity, slow movement, and gait problems. Infectious diseases such as Creutzfeldt–Jakob disease or AIDS can also cause dementia. Due to deterioration of the cerebrospinal fluid system, there is a possibility of normal pressure hydrocephalus, which can occur with people who tend to develop after a head injury. The symptoms of this are dementia, incontinence, and gait disturbances.

Ginkgo biloba is commonly thought to prevent dementia and loss of cognitive function. Studies demonstrate that this supplement does not prevent or effectively treat dementia (DeKosky et al., 2008) nor does it halt cognitive function decline (Snitz et al., 2009). Most people with dementia are given a cholinesterase inhibitor such as Tacrine (Cognex), Donepezil (Aricept), or Glalantamine (Reminyl) with the latter two most common because they can be administered only once a day. There is also a glutamate antagonist, memantine (Namenda), that has had good effect in prolonging function.

Integumentary Problems, Pathophysiology, Management

Older adults are most prone to skin problems because of sun exposure or infection due to decreased immunological function, decreased circulation, and being more prone to dehydration. Therefore, as the skin ages, one can assess thinner, drier, and wrinkled skin along with a change in pigmentation owing to fewer melanocytes. The sebaceous, eccrine, and apocrine glands also atrophy so there is less secretions from each gland. Hair color changes and most individuals experience a thinning of the hair along with fewer hair follicles.

Older adults may experience *pruritius* if they have liver failure or on specific drugs or from a skin rash or lesion, or just from dry skin. In fact, itching is considered the most frequent problem of all primary skin disorders. When determining which topical corticosteroid to use, always follow "the start low and go slow" philosophy. It is important to choose the lowest potency and work-up as the effectiveness is determined. The severity, location, and any history the person has with the rash need to be determined. Older adults need to use low-potency steroids such as *Hydrocortisone* 1% as their skin tends to be thinner. If the rash is on the thick skin such as palms or soles, then a higher potency steroid will be needed such as *Triamcinolone* 0.1% for moderate problems and *Clobetasol* when a high potency steroid is needed. Note also that ointments are more potent than creams, which are stronger than lotions. If a fungal infection is suspected, avoid steroids because the steroid will most likely worsen the infection. Generally, a demonstration if possible of the application is helpful because 0.5 g of a cream should be able to manage one adult hand's surface area, so this is a sparing application. If there is no dermatitis or lesion, then the nurse practitioner needs to rule out metabolic problems with blood work and make appropriate referrals. Xerosis or dry skin is common among older adults and needs to be prevented and/ or managed with emollients and good hydration. Bacterial infections such as staphylococcus aureus or MRSA and group A or C hemolytic streptococci are most frequent. Appropriate antibiotics such as cephalexin (Keflex) or doxycycline are used.

Older adults can also acquire fungal infections with the most frequent being *tinea*, caused by a dermatophyte, which can occur in the scalp, between the toes, the nails, on the torso, and the groin. There are several antifungal treatments, but Clotrimazole (Canesten) is very commonly used. Crusting lesions tend most frequently to be caused by *tinea*. Fungal infections also occur in the nail plate of both the hands and feet and are referred to as tinea unguium or onychomycosis. Paronychia is a fungal infection of the cuticle.

Bacterial infections of the skin such as staphylococcus aureus cause *folliculitis,* which are infected hair follicles. Generally, good hygiene with the use of a shaving cream with aloe or some sensitive skin emollient will prevent a recurrence; however, an antibiotic may be needed. *Furuncles or boils* are also caused by staphylococcus aureus and are more serious infected hair follicles that will need an antibiotic such as Cephalexin (Keflex). A more serious skin infection are *carbuncles*, which are a collection of infected hair follicles and often an abscess forms which will need an incision and drainage and possibly an intravenous antibiotic. It will be important to assess for MRSA with each of these infections.

Yeast is responsible for *candidiasis* infections which are frequently seen with older adults who have poor hygiene, diabetes, take prolonged antibiotic therapy, are immunocompromised, or are obese. Individuals with skin folds are prone to *candidiasis intertrigo* and need to try to prevent this by keeping these areas dry and clean. If the patient is not able to keep the skin fold areas dry when they have this fungal infection, then the nurse practitioner may need to order Nystatin cream BID for approximately 10 days. Candida also is found frequently in the vagina and oral cavity and will need treatment with antifungals such as Diflucan (Fluconazole) for vaginal candidiasis and Nystatin for thrush.

Herpes zoster is seen in all ages but more frequently in older adults and must be managed aggressively with antiviral medications to avoid postherpetic neuralgia. This vesicular rash begins as erythema, is painful, and manifests in a linear pattern along a dermatome. The vaccine, Zostavax, is recommended to prevent herpes zoster for adults above 60 years. It is thought to reduce the extent in some and in 51% actually prevent shingles and/or postherpetic neuralgia. Some side effects of the vaccine are headache and discomfort at the injection site. Postherpetic neuralgia is extremely painful, and individuals will need capsaicin (Zostrix) cream or the use of cool compresses to relieve some of the discomfort. It takes many weeks for the pain to be relieved, and for some, it is a very uncomfortable sensation for a lengthy amount of time. Primary and secondary skin lesions are commonly seen on older adults, which can be papular (raised) or macular (non-raised). A nodule is a papule more than 5 mm in size.

Atopic dermatitis is a result of an allergic response to some allergen such as copper or silver or a component of soap or shampoo or perhaps an exposure to poison ivy or sumac. It generally looks erythematous, causes pruritis, can swell, and have vesicular lesions. It is necessary to determine the trigger of the allergic response and remove it to prevent recurrence. Generally, whenever the person is exposed to the specific antigen, an erythematous inflammatory rash will develop, but it will be a varying manifestation at each occurrence. Steroidal creams are therapeutic and stop the itching. *Contact dermatitis* occurs when an individual has contact with a mineral such as lead or silver on a watch or jewelry and manifests an erythematous randomly patterned rash. Sometimes, people with specific occupations such as jeweler or chemist develop contact dermatitis to elements they come in contact with frequently in the work setting. Seborrheic dermatitis is seen with older adults often in the scalp, around eyebrows and eyelids, in the ear canals, and nasolabial folds. It appears as yellowish or tan scaly plaque. Emollients and good hygiene can prevent this dermatitis from recurrence.

Benign Lesions—Senile lentigos are normal findings with older adults. Skin tags also known as acrochordons are benign papillomas often found on the trunk, neck, or under the breast in older people. Also seborrheic keratoses are also seen with age and are benign greasy, wart-like and "stuck on" lesions found on the extremities, neck, and shoulders. They can range in size from 1–2 mm to 5 cm and are normally the individual's skin color or sometimes very dark. Both of these benign lesions will not become malignant but can be cauterized to improve physical appearance.

Verruca or *warts* are rough papules caused by human papillomavirus often found on feet or hands and can be removed with cryotherapy.

Premalignant Lesions—The most frequent growth that can become malignant is actinic keratosis, which are papules that are light to dark colored that appear in sun-exposed areas of the skin. A skin biopsy can assist in diagnosing these lesions that should be removed by cryotherapy or pharmacologic management because they can progress to squamous cell carcinoma.

Malignant Lesions—Basal cell carcinomas are firm papules with umbilicated centers that tend to be pearly in color and arise on sun-exposed areas of the skin. Depending on the size and cytology of the tissue removed with biopsy, Mohs cryotherapy or radiotherapy will be used or the tissue will be surgically removed. *Squamous* cell lesions will often be rough, scaly, and reddened and will be opaque nodules seen on sun-exposed areas of the skin. Similar treatment as basal cell carcinoma will remove the squamous cell cancer growths. Squamous cell carcinoma is more likely to metastasize than basal cell cancer. *Melanoma* often occurs in individuals who have had extensive sun damage and is a malignant lesion with melanocytes. The ABCD rule is a good tool to use to identify suspicious lesions that may be melanoma and includes assessing for asymmetry, irregular borders, color, and diameter of lesion. An oncologist will manage melanoma with chemotherapy, surgery, radiation, and immunotherapy.

Psoriasis has scaling, sliver-colored lesions and is a difficult to manage problem for some patients. It is a proliferative skin disorder with epidermal cell turnover every 3 to 4 days. Using calcitriol (vectical) ointment for mild to moderate plaque psoriasis has been successful. This ointment is a vitamin D analog that has antiproliferative and immunomodulating action (Lehmann, 2009). It may be necessary to add a steroid such as Clobetasol (Temovate) or Halobetasol (Ultravate) as an initial treatment and then titrate down as the psoriasis becomes more manageable or a referral to a dermatologist may be warranted (Greenberg, 2008).

Lichen planus is another papulosquamous skin disorder that causes inflammation of the mucous membranes and skin. Generally, it presents as purple, nonscaling small lesions on the wrists, ankles, and genitalia. It does cause severe drying of the area involved and can be pruritic.

Rosacea is common with older adults and is manifested by red papules or plaques with telangiectasia around the face, specifically the nose, cheeks, and chin. People should avoid the sun and generally use Retin A to decrease the redness.

Pressure ulcers occur frequently on immobilized older adults on the sacrum or any bony prominence that is adherent to the bed. Due to the high pressure on the skin surface exceeding the skin capillary pressure of 25 mmHg, the blood vessels are occluded so that the surrounding tissue becomes anoxic and creates an ulcer.

Wounds present challenges to the primary care provider who must make sound decisions as to whether to manage them or refer. For example, an individual with a facial laceration will require sutures and should be seen by a plastic surgeon. Someone who needs one suture in the back of the neck at the hairline could be more adequately sutured in the primary care clinic. If the individual has a large wound that needs incision and drainage, a surgeon is most appropriate for managing the wound. Steri-strips are used for superficial lacerations only. If the older adult with a wound presents and complain of having contact with metal, then the provider needs to administer a tetanus injection if the individual has not had one in 5 years. If the older adult has not had a T-dap, then they should receive one injection of DTaP with subsequent tetanus boosters every 10 years or when needed. This is due to the potential of acquiring pertussis.

Sensory Problems, Pathophysiology, Management—Older adults are prone to sensory loss as they age. Hearing, smell, and vision are among the most frequent problem areas.

Due to decreased circulation, slowed basal metabolic rate, more sedentary lifestyle, and decreased vasoconstrictor and vasodilator ability, older adults have poor responses to environmental temperature changes. They also have a difficult time manifesting a fever with an elevated temperature when exposed to inflammation or infection.

Cataracts are common in older adults and are a result of clouding of the lens. Generally, people complain of blurred vision especially at night and see halo images around lights along with decreased visual acuity. The rule of thumb is that when symptoms of cataracts impact an individual's activities of daily life, it is time for surgery, which is the only treatment. Diabetes mellitus, smoking, genetics, use of steroids, and alcohol can cause cataracts to form. *Glaucoma* is also more common with older adults and is caused by increased intraocular pressure which will gradually compress the optic nerve and cause loss of peripheral vision and decrease visual acuity. People with ocular hypertension, diabetes mellitus, myopia, steroid use, and hypertensive crises are more apt to have glaucoma. There are different types of glaucoma, and the more common type with older adults occurs slowly and is called open angle glaucoma, which in most cases the person is unaware. A more acute onset of eye pain, eye redness, headache, nausea, and decreased vision is less common and is called primary angle closure glaucoma. *Macular degeneration* is also more frequently seen with older adults, which decreases the central vision since it is caused by multiple hemorrhages in the retina which are manifested by a gray spot/shadow in the central eye causing decreased visual acuity and gradually will leave the individual with mostly peripheral vision. The major cause of decreased vision with adults above 60 is age-related macular degeneration, which is a result of increased oxidative stress and capillary injury often caused by cigarette smoking, hypertension, and insulin resistance. Older adults sometimes also have a white circle at the edge of the cornea, which is a normal aging process called arcus senilis that does not impair vision.

Bacterial or viral conjunctivitis is more apt to occur with older adults with decreased cognition who might be touching their eyes or be in a long-term facility. Generally, the bacterial type causes thick yellow discharge, which especially upon awakening has "glued the eyelids together" and needs to have a wet compress applied to detach the lids. The usual treatment is Tobramycin (Tobrex) 1 gtt OU q 4 hours while awake. If the individual cannot tolerate eye drops, using Erythromycin ointment q 4 hours while awake is also effective. For individuals experiencing seasonal allergies, eye dryness and itchiness are common. Most people will have effect from taking an oral antihistamine, but one needs to assess the other medications the person may be taking to be sure that no adverse drug reactions occur. Any individual presenting to a primary care practice with loss of vision, changes in papillary response, or eye pain warrant an immediate opthamologist referral.

Hearing with older adults tends to decrease, but one of the main reasons is reversible and that is cerumen impaction due to a decrease in cerumen glands. This problem can be easily identified, and ear irrigations and demulsification medication such as Debrox can be used to prevent recurrence. Older adults are prone to *presbycusis* as they age. They are more likely to have sensorineural nonconductive problems with their hearing. *Presbycusis*, a sensorineural hearing loss of high-frequency sounds, is the most frequent hearing problem experienced by older adults and is due to degeneration of the cochlea, cranial nerve VIII, and the CNS. Symptoms tend to be insidious and progressive and occur bilaterally. It is possible that cerumen removal may correct this dysfunction. The less common hearing loss is due to blockage of sounds by the tympanic membrane and middle ear and is called conductive hearing loss. Hearing aids can assist in improving hearing for these conditions.

Older adults experience loss of olfactory sensory neurons and olfactory bulb cell degeneration, thus possibly impacting appetite and food selection (Kovacs, 2004).

For older adults who are bedridden, they will have increased risk for pressure sores and because of their decreased sensory ability, they will not be cognizant of the discomfort, so these pressure sores may magnify unnecessarily before they are identified.

More than half of older adults over 65 years have sleep disorders that may not be correlated to aging. Symptoms such as loud snoring, periods of apnea, frequent awakening during the night, and awakening due to anxiety need to be followed up and managed. Due to medications they have taken, multiple comorbidities, and changes of aging such as decreased cortisol and growth hormone, older adults are predisposed to sleep disorders. There is a correlation of sleep apnea and cardiovascular disorders (Bliwise, Ansari, Straight, & Parker, 2005).

Renal and Urologic Problems, Pathophysiology, Management

With previously ambulatory older adults who experience a fall, the nurse practitioner should rule out urosepsis and do a routine urinalysis and metabolic panel because it is common for older adults with a UTI to have mental status changes, which increases their chance for a fall. Additionally, an older adult who develops acute delirium should be checked for urosepsis.

Overactive bladder is defined as a group of symptoms including urgency, polyuria (~8 times/24 hours), and nocturia (2 times/night) in the absence of pathologic conditions (International Incontinence Society, 2010). Urinary incontinency can happen to anyone but is more prevalent with older adults. It is a severe problem that in some cases can be reversed. The two most significant factors causing increased bladder pressure, which then becomes higher than the pressure in the urethra and leak out, are (1) the detrusor muscle tone is greatly decreased if the person is taking muscle relaxants, anticholinergic drugs, or drugs causing beta adrenergic stimulation and (2) intra-abdominal pressure, which can be increased if the individual is jogging, coughing, or sneezing which ultimately causes increased bladder pressure and hence urine leakage. The most common urinary incontinence is detrusor muscle instability. The remaining four types of incontinence include overflow, functional, stress, and iatrogenic, and all need to be worked up and managed. Women may have severe pelvic organ prolapsed, which will add to the incontinence. Table 5.1 describes each type of incontinence.

Patients with multiple neurological diseases such as a cerebrovascular accident (CVA), spinal cord injury (SCI), and multiple sclerosis (MS) with neurogenic bladders may have detrusor dysfunction that causes incontinence.

TABLE 5.1

Incontinence, Pathophysiology, and Manifestations

Incontinence Category	Description	Pathophysiology	Examples of Manifestations
Overflow	Leaking of urine caused by forces exerted on the over-distended bladder	The bladder has lost its tone or a mechanical force is exerting pressure on the bladder causing the leakage	Frequency, urgency, nocturia, and constant dribbling
Urge	Inability to stop urinating when bladder is full	The detrusor muscle is hyperactive or there is CNS dysfunction	Inability to make it to the bathroom
Stress	Loss of urine when there is increased abdominal pressure	Urethral sphincter tone is decreased and/or pelvic muscles and bladder outlet strength is weak	Running, jumping, and coughing causes urine leakage
Functional	Due to cognitive or physical dysfunction	Cognitive and mental status changes and/or physical impairment	Not able to physically get to the bathroom when desired

Older adults are more apt to develop malignancy but renal cancer is rare. Bladder cancer is more frequently seen and is caused by multiple environmental factors such as cigarette smoking, working with chemicals and toxic substances, or in the dry cleaner business. Hematuria is a significant complaint that needs thorough follow-up for it could indicate bladder cancer, renal stones, or uterine pathology.

Older adults are often infected with *Escherichia coli* or *Staphylococcus saprophyticus* because of poor hygiene or incontinence and then are frequently diagnosed with a urinary tract infection (UTI). Often, they are given two antibiotics if they are hospitalized due to the usual culprit, gram-negative bacteria, and develop urosepsis. They are prescribed ampicillin (Omnipen) and Gentamicin as the first choice. Other risk factors that increase their chance of acquiring a UTI are a foley catheterization or being institutionalized. If they have a positive MRSA infection, they will be given Vancomycin. If they are Vancomycin sensitive or resistant, they will be given Synercid (Quinupristin) or Zyvox (Linezolid). Men will have more chance of acquiring a UTI if they have prostate enlargement, and occasionally older adults have urethral strictures, which will obstruct urine flow causing retrograde flow and a UTI. Older adults have more risk of developing a complicated UTI because they have more possibility of the aforementioned issues. An uncomplicated UTI is generally because of E. coli invasion and can be managed similarly to outpatients with UTIs. Depending on the variable involved, the provider can prescribe Bactrim, Nitrofurantoin (Macrobid), or Ciprofloxacin (Cipro) for 3 to 5 days to 7 days.

The BUN of older adults reduces with age to a normal range of 10 to 20 mg/dL, and this should be used as a benchmark along with serum creatinine to assess renal function. Older adults with heart failure gradually have decreased cardiac output, and this is manifested in several ways among these being a lower urine output. The patient may not be aware of the decrease as it is generally an insidious process, but if the individual experiences acute heart failure, they may be knowledgeable. Older adults taking diuretics for heart failure or hypertension can develop hypokalemia/hyperkalemia depending on the stage of renal disease, postural hypotension, worsening renal function as evidenced by positive proteinuria or left ventricular hypertrophy. Any individual with known renal insufficiency or failure cannot take thiazide diuretics and will have to use loop diuretics if they need diuresis.

Nephrotic syndrome with adults can occur secondary to conditions such as diabetes, amyloidosis, and lupus erythematosus. It indicates massive leakage of proteins from the glomerular membrane. This condition can also be due to certain drugs, infections, and malignancies. Generally, there is a 1:1 ratio of protein to creatinine.

Older adults with long-term diabetes, liver disease, or overuse of NSAIDs will also have nephropathy that will gradually increase, and it is not uncommon for the patient to be diagnosed with chronic renal failure. A good indicator of renal disease is microalbuminuria that develops slowly as the glomerular basement membrane deteriorates. Renal failure is divided into five stages with Stage 1 = an increase in plasma creatinine and BUN and normal glomerular filtration rate (GFR), which for older adults is ~90 mL/minute; Stage 2 = decreased GFR 60 to 89 mL/minute, increased creatinine and BUN and positive protein in urine, Stage 3 = decreased GFR 30 to 59 with gradually increasing BUN, creatinine, and positive protein, Stage 4 = severe decrease in GFR to 15 mL/min. with increasing other parameters, and Stage 5 = GFR less than 15 mL/min. Approximately 80% of the nephrons will no longer be able to function when an individual begins to manifest signs and symptoms of end stage renal disease in chronic renal failure. This is generally an insidious process of renal insufficiency proceeding to dysfunction and then to renal failure where dialysis or a renal transplant is needed. Symptoms include fatigue, pruritis, swelling, nausea, vomiting, decreased urine output, cognitive changes, and signs of potassium, sodium, calcium, and phosphorous electrolyte imbalance. Chronic renal failure (CRF) causes an irreversible loss of renal function, which will ultimately impact all body systems as it evolves into end-stage renal disease (ESRD). Table 5.2, Complications of Chronic Renal Failure, illustrates the organ system and common manifestations of CRF.

Older adults may be prone to developing renal stones because they are often more immobile and over time stones form especially in the ureters. Generally, they complain of costovertebral angle tenderness (CVA)

TABLE 5.2

Complications of Chronic Renal Failure

Organ System	Examples of Manifestations
Musculoskeletal	Bone fractures and osteodystrophy
Cardiopulmonary	Increased BP, pluritis, and pericarditis
Neurological	Drowsiness, neuropathy, depression, and insomnia
Endocrine	Fatigue, lack of energy, insulin resistance, and hypothyroidism
Reproductive	Impotence and decreased libido
Hematological	Anemia and fatigue
Dermatological	Uremic frost, pruritis, and brittle and dry hair
Gastro-intestinal	Nausea, vomiting, and uremic fetor

and colic-like cramping pain. They may also have a decreased urine output because of the stone obstruction. They need to have an adequate fluid intake and, in some cases, NSAIDs to relieve the discomfort as they try to pass the stone. If the stone is not passed they will need lithroscopic surgery to remove the stone(s).

Glomerular disorders can occur with older adults and can manifest as sudden or insidious elevations of BP, swelling, and increased serum creatinine and blood urea nitrogen. Because of the increased permeability of the glomerular capillary, proteins will be excreted in the urine, which will cause fluid in the vascular bed to seep out and cause edema. Some older adults may have a toxic reaction to diagnostic contrast dye or medications that can cause glomerulonephritis, which is a type of acute renal failure. Hematuria, proteinuria, and low-urine output will possibly be evident if measured, but generally, no symptoms are manifested until the glomerular filtration rate (GFR) is decreased by half. If a creatinine clearance is performed, the flow will most likely be less than 75 ml/minute. Older adults may need to have lower dosages of drugs due to decreased creatinine clearance, which they may experience if they have renal insufficiency (GFR is decreased by 25%). Even with normal blood urea nitrogen and serum creatinine, they still may have decreased creatinine clearance which would be less than 75 ml/minute. The rule of thumb is to halve all dosages of older adults with abnormal BUN and serum creatinine because the predicted creatinine clearance will be less than 50 ml/minute. A formula often used to estimate the creatinine clearance is CrCl = 140 minus the person's age multiplied by person's weight in kgs divided by serum creatinine multiplied by 72 and then for women the result of the above formula is multiplied by 0.85.

Benign prostate hyperplasia is common with the majority of older men above 65 years. The enlargement of the prostate is a concern when it grows big enough to compress the urethra. Many men are on alpha blockers to decrease the lower urinary tract symptoms such as nocturia and frequency. All older men should have a prostate-specific antigen (PSA) drawn annually and more frequently if they have any risks for this cancer. The normal range for PSA is 0.4–4.0 ng/dL but can be considered normal for older men up to 6.0 ng/dL. The lower the PSA, the lesser the chance of prostate cancer; however, men can have prostate cancer and a normal PSA. It is most significant that older men have annual PSA screening and any change from the individual's normal PSA can be followed up. Often with older men who are diagnosed with low-grade disease and a low PSA, the active surveillance management is recommended because of the potential complications post-prostatectomy. Unfortunately, *prostate cancer* rarely has any symptoms until it has reached advanced stages. Men with benign prostate hyperplasia may experience some urinary obstruction with the enlarged prostate compressing the urethra that could cause postrenal acute renal failure. They may be candidates for prostatectomy to relieve the urinary obstruction.

Reproductive Problems, Pathophysiology, Management

Older adults are at risk for sexually transmitted infections (STI) and need to be assessed similar to others. The most common diseases tested include *Gonorrhea, Chlamydia, Syphilis, HIV,* and *HPV.* Using the Center for Disease Control 2006 STI Guidelines, one can easily manage these problems with recommended pharmacological interventions. Access is available at *www .cdc.gov/std/treatment.*

Male Reproductive Disorders with older adults tend to include penile rashes such as scabies lichen planus, scabies, and psoriasis and have similar management as younger adults. *Fungal* infections of the scrotum are common with men in long-term care and need to be assessed and treated with Nystatin. Redness around the genital area but not the scrotum generally indicates tinea cruris. A *hydrocele* is common and presents as a painless unilateral swelling of fluid that transilluminates through the scrotal sac and is most easily visualized anterior to the testis. It is caused by scrotal swelling secondary to increased fluid within the tunica vaginalis (Williams, 2008). A *varicocele,* caused by inadequate valves in the spermatic veins, tends to cause some alarm in the patient because it feels like a "bag of worms" and most likely is on the left side. If the varicocele is on the right side, it is more likely malignant and a more serious etiology and will need to be seen by a urologist.

Men can have some degree of low libido depending on what type of chronic disease they may have. Male sexual dysfunction such as erectile dysfunction can be due to a myriad of issues such as having diabetes mellitus or renal failure or from medications such as selective serotonin reuptake inhibitors (SSRIs), statins, tricyclic antidepressants, and calcium channel blockers. Often, oral phosphodiesterase inhibitors such as Sildenafil (Viagra), Vardenafil (Levitra), and Tadalafil (Cialis) are prescribed as first line of action. Men are more apt to have erectile dysfunction from these aforementioned conditions and advanced age above 85 years than a decreased testosterone level that is a part of normal aging.

Men who are in long-term care facilities may have *balanitis*, which is redness of the foreskin caused by an increased amount of smegma under the foreskin or *phimosis* which is foreskin that cannot be retracted. It is essential that the older male receives good hygiene to the genital area and be assessed consistently. Men are more prone to breast cancer after the age of 60, so they should be assessed more frequently if there is a known risk factor.

Female Reproductive–Abnormal uterine bleeding with older women signals possible malignancy, and this needs to be fully worked up by a gynecologist. *Endometrial cancer* is more likely to occur and will require a dilation and curettage so that the uterine lining can be tested. Other cancers that are seen with older women are ovarian and breast. A frequent benign tumor that needs to be assessed for size is the uterine fibroid or leiomyoma, which are benign smooth muscle tumors in the myometrium. Pelvic and vaginal ultrasound testing will assist in diagnosing the individual. They may need to be surgically removed if they cause uterine bleeding, pain, or other symptoms related to the pressure they may be having on the bladder, for example.

Most women are in menopause around 51 to 52 years of age, but they may have other variables impacting them, so it is wise to assess an older woman's hormone profile especially for follicle-stimulating hormone (FSH). Follow-up is advised so that two positive FSH tests are determined before saying someone is in or postmenopausal. Most women in menopause experience severe hot flashes, which are correlated with imbalances of leutinizing hormone (LH). Black Cohosh, a complementary supplement, is the only herb associated with decreasing hot flashes. The other major vasomotor symptom is night sweats, which impacts sleep and may cause irritability or other mood fluctuations (Moore, 2010). There is much controversy over the most therapeutic and safe management of the moderate to severe vasomotor response symptoms, but the general guideline is to administer the smallest dose for the shortest time and to insure that the patient has been told the benefits and risks of hormone therapy (Moore, 2010). Urogenital symptoms such as dryness, irritation, and discomfort with urination tend to occur approximately 2 years after menopause (Allmen & Moore, 2010). The vaginal atrophy causing dyspareunia secondary to decreased estrogen and the irritating UTIs due to the increased pH of the vagina are part of the vulvavaginal atrophy that many older women experience. Management for these symptoms includes nonhormonal lubricants and moisturizers. It is not recommended to prescribe hormonal therapy for these symptoms unless the individual also suffers from moderate to severe vasomotor response symptoms (Allmen & Moore, 2010).

Women need to be assessed yearly for sexually transmitted infections (STIs) if they are sexually active and not to assume older adults are not sexually active. *Pelvic inflammatory disease* is possible if the STI or other microbe is not identified and managed. There are older women who have human papilloma virus (HPV), which could become cervical cancer depending on the type and needs to be consistently managed to prevent the cancer from occurring. *Vaginal candidiasis* is experienced by many women post use of an antibiotic or if they are not able to keep their genital area dry and clean. Some older women develop a highly sensitive vulvar region and continuously have inflamed external genitalia and need expert hygiene and possibly pharmacologic management. Bacterial vaginitis is another frequent infection for some older women who may need assistance in developing a vaginal hygiene protocol.

Older adults sometimes need assistance with increasing libido that may be decreased due to a medication they may be taking, for example, an antidepressant such as an SSRI. Lack of estrogen may be causing dyspareunia, which can be supplemented with a minute amount of topical estrogen before intercourse.

As women age, they are more vulnerable to develop *cystoceles, uterine prolapse*, and *rectoceles*. Annual exams can identify this muscular and fascia tissue loss so that appropriate referrals and management can be implemented.

All breast changes need follow-up in older women, both nonproliferative lesions such as fibrocystic breast disease and proliferative breast lesions, to determine if they are benign or malignant. Breast cancer is the second most common killer after lung cancer.

Geropsychiatric Problems, Pathophysiology, Management

Older adults are often experiencing some type of sadness, but some are definitely depressed and should be seen by a psychiatric specialist if symptoms do not improve after 4 weeks. Sometimes, the most significant manifestation is when an older adult complains of severe fatigue and always makes an excuse such as "I am too tired to do anything, you go ahead with the kids and I will see you another time." There are depression scales and other measurement tools that can assist the primary care provider in determining if referral is needed for appropriate intervention for mental health diagnoses. Major depressive disorder is defined as the individual experiencing at least five symptoms including feeling sad most of the day everyday over a 2-week period. The provider must give careful attention to medicating older adults with depression as the antidepressants have multiple side effects such as decreased libido, difficulty sleeping, nausea, and agitation. Cognitive behavioral therapy may be a first action to assist older adults with managing their depression. If the person does seem to require a medication, the first drug category to use is the SSRIs. Although it is recommended to avoid fluoxetine (Prozac) with older adults, it has such a long half-life. Monoamine oxidase inhibitors and tricyclic antidepressants are also used for depression. All three drug categories will take some time for a response to be noted so other therapy needs to also be in place. The newer antipsychotic agents are less likely to cause extrapyramidal effects versus the conventional antipsychotics with older adults. For older adults who are in a vegetative state from depression, use of electroshock therapy may be effective. Often, if the depression is eliminated, the person's confusion or even dementia will resolve. Many older adults with depression will have other comorbidities, so it is important to refer to a psychiatrist or psychiatric nurse practitioner regarding management. They should be scheduled to see the therapist at least every 2 weeks initially for therapy and not just given medications. Individuals with recurrent depression that is more than 3 episodes of depression should have long-term therapy with a psychiatric provider.

Anxiety disorders are another common geropsychiatric disorder and can occur after an episode of depression. Older adults can experience panic attacks, obsessive–compulsive disorder, acute stress, and post-traumatic stress disorder. General anxiety disorder is diagnosed if the individual has had 6 months of excessive worrying. Also the primary care provider can screen older adults for alcoholism with the CAGE tool and also test for substance abuse. These individuals should be referred to a psychiatric nurse practitioner or a psychiatrist for appropriate therapy and possible medication management.

Domestic violence is common with elders and needs to be identified by primary care providers because they probably see the victim most frequently. When individuals present with physical complaints but no pathology is found, the provider should follow up on the possibility of domestic violence. Because of the prevalence of domestic violence, it is important to discuss violence with the patient similar to discussing the importance of wearing a seat belt at all times when riding in a car. One could bring the domestic violence topic up by stating a fact such as violence is more common today than ever before, and it often plays a role in many relationships such as with a spouse, child, grandchild, brother or sister, or significant other. When a victim of domestic violence is significant, other person does all of the talking for the victim and insists on being with the patient at all times; the provider should be more vigilant in screening for domestic violence.

REFERENCES

Adelman, J. U., Adelman, L. C., Freeman, M. C., Von Seggern, R. L., Drake, J. (2004). Cost considerations of acute migraine treatment. *Headache, 44*, 271–285.

Ahmed, N., Mandel, R., & Fain, M. J. (2007). Frailty: An emerging geriatric syndrome. *The American Journal of Medicine, 120*(9), 748–753.

Allmen, T., & Moore, A. (2010). Attention and intervention: Responding to vaginal changes of menopause. *Women's Health Care: A Practical Journal for Nurse Practitioners, 5*(9), 39–52.

American Diabetes Association. (2009). *American Diabetes Association's New Clinical Practice Recommendations Promote A1C as Diagnostic Test for Diabetes.* Retrieved May 6, 2010, from http://www.diabetes.org/for-media/2009/cpr-2010-a1c-diagnostic-tool.html

Andreoli, T., Benjamin, I., Griggs, R., & Wing, E. (2010). *Andreoli and Carpenter's Cecil essentials of medicine* (8th ed.). St. Louis: Saunders.

Bliwise, D. L., Ansari, F. P., Straight, L. B., & Parker, K. P. (2005). Age changes in timing and 24 hour distribution of self-reported sleep. *American Journal of Geriatric Psychiatry, 13*(12), 1077–1082.

Burke, M., & Laramie, J. (2004). *Primary care of the older adult: A multidisciplinary approach.* St. Louis, MO: Mosby.

Capezuti, E., Zwicker, D, Mezey, M., & Fulmer, T. (Eds.). (2008). *Evidence based geriatric nursing protocols for best practice* (3rd ed.). New York: Springer Publishing.

Cherniak, E. P., Levis, S., & Troen, B. (2008). Hypovitaminosis D: A stealthy epidemic that requires treatment. *Geriatrics, 63*(4), 26–30.

Chowdhury, B. A., & Dal Pan, G. (2010). The FDA and safe use of long-acting beta-agonists in the treatment of asthma. *New England Journal of Medicine, 362*(13), 1169–1171.

DeKosky, S. T., Wiliamson, J. D., Fitzpatrick, A. L., Kronmal, R. A., Ives, D. G., Saxton, J. A., et al. (2008). Ginkgo biloba for prevention of dementia: A randomized controlled trial. *Journal of American Medical Association, 300*(19), 2253–2262.

Edmunds, M. W., & Mayhew, M. S. (2009). *Pharmacology for the primary care provider* (3rd ed.). St. Louis, MO: Elsevier.

Greenberg, R. (2008). A short course in topical psoriasis agents. *The Clinical Advisor, 7*, 23–24, 25.

Gueldner, S., Grabo, T., Newman, E., & Cooper, D. (2008). *Osteoporosis: Clinical guidelines for prevention, diagnosis, and management.* New York: Springer Publishers.

Hensley, R., & Williams, A. (2010). Clinical coach for nurse practitioners. Philadelphia: F. A. Davis.

International Incontinence Society. (2010). *Overactive Bladder and Incontinence Guidelines.* Retrieved May 22, from http://www.medscape.com/viewarticle/582646_4

Kovacs, T. (2004). Mechanisms of olfactory dysfunction in aging and neurodegenerative disorders. *Ageing Research Reviews, 3*(2), 215–232.

Luthy, K. E., Peterson, N. E., & Wilkinson, J. (2008). Cost-efficient treatment options for uninsured or underinsured patients for five common conditions. *The Journal for Nurse Practitioners* (8), 577–584.

Lehmann, B. (2009). Role of the vitamin D3 pathway in health and diseased skin—facts, contradictions and hypotheses. *Experimental Dermatology, 18*(2), 97–108.

Mayo Clinic. (2010). *HIV: Tests and diagnosis.* Retrieved on May 7, 2010, from http://www.mayoclinic.com/health/hiv-aids/ds00005/dsection=tests-and-diagnosis

Moore, A. (2010). Bioidentical hormone therapy: What practitioners need to know now. *Women's Health Care: A Practical Journal for Nurse Practitioners, 5*(9), 10–18.

Mayhew, Ms. (2009). Vitamin D deficiency and treatment. *The Journal for Nurse Practitioners, 5*(10), 773–774.

Morris, S., Van Swol, M., & Udani, B. (2005). The less familiar side of heart failure: Symptomatic diastolic dysfunction. *The Journal of Family Practice, 54*(6), 501–511.

National Heart Lung and Blood Institute (2004). Third Report of the Expert Panel on Detection, Evaluation, and Treatment of High Blood cholesterol in Adults. Retrieved November 11, 2010, from http://www.nhlbi.nih.gov/guidelines/cholesterol/index.htm

National Heart, Lung, & Blood Institute (2007). *Guidelines for Treatment of Asthma.* Retrieved March 25, 2010, from http://www.nhlbi.nih.gov/guidelines/asthma

[7th] Report of the Joint National Committee on Prevention, Detection, Evaluation, and Treatment of Blood Pressure (JNC 7) 2004 Retrieved May 11, 2010, from http://www.nhlbi.nih.gov/guidelines/hypertension/phycard.pdf

Ryan, P. J. (2007). Vitamin D therapy in clinical practice: One dose does not fit all. *International Journal of Clinical Practice, 61*(11), 1894–1899.

Snitz, B. E., O'Meara, E. S., Carlson, M. C., Arnold, A. M., Ives, D. G., Rapp, S. R., et al. (2009). Ginkgo biloba for preventing cognitive decline in older adults: A randomized trial. *Journal of American Medical Association, 302*(24), 2663–2670.

Syroney, L., & Franjesevic, A. (2010). Vitamin D deficiency: Screening and treatment in primary care. *Advance for Nurse Practitioners, 5*, 37–40.

TB Elimination: Diagnosis of TB Disease. CDC. (2009). Retrieved April 1, 2010, from CDC guidelines available at http://www.cdc.gov/tb/publications/PDF/1376.pdf

United States Food & Drug Administration Agency. (2008). *Fluoroquinolone Antimicrobial Drugs.* Retrieved on March 3, 2010, from http://www.fda.gov/Safety/MedWatch/SafetyInformation/SafetyAlertsforHumanMedicalProducts/ucm089652.htm

U. S. Preventive Services. *Task Force* (2010). *Guidelines for Care.* Retrieved May 20, 2010, from http://www.ahrq.gov/clinic/uspstfix.htm

Williams, M. (2008). *Geriatric physical diagnosis: A guide to observation and assessment.* Jefferson, NC: McFarland & Company, Publishers.

TEST QUESTIONS

1. The most frequent etiology of pain for older people is generally because of one of the following:

   A. Inflammatory and infectious processes

   B. Musculoskeletal and peripheral vascular disease

   C. Cancer and peripheral vascular disease

   D. Cardiovascular disease and inflammation

2. The World Health Organization (WHO) recommends the use of three-step analgesic ladder when deciding on pain management. In order of first choice to second to third choice, the following drug categories are used:

   A. NSAIDs, nonopioids, and opioids

   B. Nonopioids, opioid antagonists, and opioids

   C. Nonopioids, opioids, and adjuvant agents

   D. NSAIDs, opioids, and adjuvant agents

3. Analgesic drugs that should not be used for older people include Meperidine (Demerol), Propoxyphene (Darvon), Ketorolac (Toradol), and Pentazocine (Talwin) because of

   A. Sedating effects

   B. Anticholinergic effects

   C. Cardiovascular effects

   D. Central nervous system effects

4. An older adult is at higher risk to experience adverse drug events. An example of pharmacodynamic problems includes

   A. A change in sensitivity to medications

   B. Decreased renal clearance

   C. Increased amount of albumin

   D. Decreased drug-metabolizing enzymes

5. Older adults on Digoxin (Lanoxin) should not be prescribed the following antibiotic because of a high possibility of acquiring digoxin toxicity:

    A. Erythromycin (Ery –Tab)

    B. Clarithromycin (Biaxin)

    C. Azithromycin (Z-pak)

    D. Doxycycline (Doryx)

6. Mrs. Smith, an 81-year-old patient on Warfarin (Coumadin) in your primary care clinic, requests that she have an additional over-the-counter medication to assist her in "feeling her best." She should be told that the following herbal remedies interact with her Warfarin:

    A. St. John's Wart and glucosamine

    B. Ginseng and Echinacea

    C. Ginkgo biloba and garlic

    D. Glucosamine and ginseng

7. Older adults are at risk for adverse drug events with antihypertensives. For example, elderly taking diuretics and alpha blockers are likely to experience

    A. Constipation

    B. Incontinence

    C. Confusion

    D. Orthostatic hypotension

8. Respiratory depression, cognitive changes, and confusion are commonly experienced by older adults taking

    A. Sedative–hypnotic agents

    B. Mood-stabilizing drugs

    C. Antipsychotic agents

    D. Anticholinergic drugs

9. Mrs. Rondu, 78 years old, has been taking Nortriptyline (Pamelor). She presents to her primary care provider with complaints of constipation, dry mouth, and a slight blurring of vision that started this morning. A rationale for these problems include one of the following:

   A. Hypothyroidism

   B. Anticholinergic side effects

   C. Dehydration

   D. Decreased liver metabolizing enzymes

10. Mr. Tormaly, 83 years old, is diagnosed with depression and is being prescribed an SSRI agent. Most likely the drug chosen will be

    A. Paroxetine (Paxil)

    B. St. John's Wart

    C. Citalopram (Celexa)

    D. Fluoxetine (Prozac)

11. The newer antipsychotic agents are less likely to cause the following side effects versus the conventional antipsychotics with older adults:

    A. Hallucinations and delusions

    B. Incontinence of stool and urine

    C. Diplopia and blurred vision

    D. Extrapyramidal effects

12. Approximately 30% of all prescriptive drugs and 40% of over-the-counter drugs are for older adults. One can easily see that it is common for older adults to be at high risk for experiencing polypharmacy. This term can best be described as follows:

    A. Having too many options to purchase drug prescriptions, so the older adult becomes confused as to the best way of obtaining one's medications

    B. Taking too many over-the-counter and prescription drugs than are clinically needed for an individual

    C. Taking too many prescription medications with the potential for multiple adverse drug reactions

    D. Having a provider prescribe too many drugs from one drug category for an older adult with a long-term chronic illness that is not responding well to the original drug or dosage

13. Delirium presents in older adults as

    A. Insidious loss of cognitive function and memory

    B. Long-term pattern of mental status changes and cognitive ability

    C. Acute cognitive dysfunction and impaired attentiveness

    D. Progressive change in the level of consciousness and confusion

14. The following are most frequently the etiology of an older adult's diagnosis of delirium:

    A. Infection, neurological, or metabolic

    B. Endocrine, musculoskeletal, or neurological

    C. Metabolic, endocrine, or cardiovascular

    D. Immunological, visual, or endocrine

15. Mrs. Togatta, 84 years old, presents with her daughter who complains the mother is more forgetful, having visual hallucinations, has a loss of words, and experiencing Parkinson-like symptoms. You suspect she has the following type of dementia:

    A. Alzheimer's dementia

    B. Dementia of Parkinson's disease

    C. Dementia of the Lewy body type

    D. Vascular dementia

16. Mr. Ryan, 74 years old, presents with an irregular pulse ranging from 100 to 120 beats/minute. He states that he never had the rapid pulse feeling before and is also experiencing shortness of breath and fatigue. Most likely this dysrhythmia is

    A. Junctional rhythm

    B. Supraventricular tachycardia

    C. Atrial fibrillation

    D. Ventricular fibrillation

17. Mrs. Bee, 69 years old, has a mild aortic stenosis and has experienced a TIA. Your action is to

    A. Refer him to a cardiologist immediately

    B. Admit to the emergency department

    C. Order Warfarin 7 mg/day with follow-up in 1 week

    D. Order carotid Doppler studies within the week

18. You are working up a 70-year-old patient who presents with a persistent INR of 4.0 and who generally has a therapeutic ranging from 2.0 to 3.0. Your best action is to order

    A. 1 to 2 mg/day for the daily Warfarin (Coumadin) dose with a follow-up lab in 1 week

    B. 5 mg/day to the daily Warfarin (Coumadin) dose with a follow-up lab in 1 week

    C. 1 aspirin 84 mg/day along with the daily Warfarin (Coumadin) dose and follow-up lab in 1 week

    D. Follow-up with lab in 1 week

19. Mr. Todd, 82 years old, takes Warfarin (Coumadin) daily for management of his atrial fibrillation. He presents to the primary care clinic with a 2-day history of acute sinusitis with PND, cough, and bilateral maxillary and facial sinus tenderness. He is afebrile. The NP prescribes the following prescription:

    A. Mucinix (Guaifenesin) with decongestant

    B. Biaxin (Clarithromycin)

    C. Doxycycline (Doryx)

    D. Cefuroxime (Ceftin)

20. Older patients with mitral valve disease or a prosthetic valve should take Warfarin (Coumadin) and maintain INR between

    A. 2.0 and 2.5 seconds

    B. 1.5 and 2.0 seconds

    C. 2.0 and 3.0 seconds

    D. 2.5 and 3.5 seconds

21. Osteopenia is diagnosed when the individual patient's bone density falls

    A. Within 1 to 2 standard deviations below the mean

    B. Within 3 standard deviations below the mean

    C. Greater or equal to 2.5 standard deviations below the mean

    D. Greater than 3 standard deviations below the mean

22. The most frequent fracture sites for older adults related to osteoporosis include

    A. Cervical vertebrae, sternum, and femur

    B. Hip, spine, and wrist

    C. Sternum, hip, and humerus

    D. Hip, femur, and tibia

23. Osteoporotic fractures of the spine leads to the following manifestations:

    A. Lordosis and pigeon chest

    B. Barrel chest and abdominal protuberance

    C. Kyphosis and decreased height

    D. Abdominal protuberance and pigeon chest

24. Z-scores are often used to interpret bone density scores of individuals so that appropriate management can be implemented. Z-scores compare bone density scores

    A. Related to the patient's age and gender to a matched population

    B. Of a fracture site to standard same fracture site scores

    C. To a gender matched young adult population

    D. To T-scores of individuals above 25 years of age.

25. An older patient in a long-term care facility is told that he or she has a positive PPD. This interpretation would be based on findings that reveal

    A. Erythema at the site of administration

    B. An induration reaction less than 5 mm

    C. Erythematous circle at the site of administration

    D. An induration reaction less than 5 mm

26. Mrs. Smith, 82 years old, presents to the emergency department with swollen feet, cough, shortness of breath, and fatigue that has been worsening over the last 3 days. The nurse practitioner includes the following in the patient's interventions after admitting her:

A. Diuretic

B. Intubation

C. EEG

D. CAT scan of head

27. Mr. Relli, 77 years old, presents to the primary care provider with rales, shortness of breath, productive cough, fever, and cold symptoms. He shares he has been ill for over 3 to 4 weeks. He has no rhonchi except in the lower left lobe where he complains of discomfort. Your first action is to

A. Order a PA and lateral chest x-ray

B. Order Mucinex to thin the bronchial secretions

C. Order an AP lateral chest x-ray

D. Refer for a bronchoscopy

28. Older women experience many symptoms with menopause largely because of decreased estrogen. The most frequent vasomotor symptoms that women will present to their primary care provider for management are as follows:

A. Vaginal itching and dyspareunia

B. Hot flashes and night sweats

C. Anxiety and palpitations

D. Dyspnea and cough

29. Due to loss of estrogen with menopause, many women experience an increase in UTIs. This is mostly because of

A. Decreased perfusion to the detrusor muscle

B. Increased vaginal cilia

C. Prolonged urinary outflow due to urethral narrowing

D. Decreased vaginal pH

30. The guideline to follow regarding prescribing for hormonal therapy to menopausal women is to

   A. Only use topical estrogen

   B. Never prescribe estrogen

   C. Prescribe estrogen at the lowest effective dose for the shortest time period only for moderate to severe vasomotor symptoms

   D. Use of estrogen for hormonal replacement therapy postmenopause is reserved for physicians only

31. Older adults with the following habits are at a higher risk of developing peptic ulcer disease or gastritis:

   A. Cigarette smoking and use of PPIs

   B. High fat diet and sedentary lifestyle

   C. Tobacco chewing and depression

   D. Cigarette smoking and NSAIDs

32. Obese older adults are at high risk for developing fatty liver disease. The following liver diseases will gradually progress to cirrhosis:

   A. Metabolic syndrome

   B. Nonalcoholic steatohepatitis

   C. Hepatitis A

   D. Nonalcoholic fatty liver disease

33. Mrs. Elba, 84 years old, has been in excellent health all of her life. She presents to the primary care provider with the following complaints which she says she never experienced before now: left-sided abdominal discomfort, increased flatulence, and patterns of diarrhea, and constipation. Your differential includes the following diagnosis:

   A. GERD

   B. Crohn's disease

   C. Diverticulitis

   D. Cholecystitis

Older adults with RA, AIDS, systemic lupus erythematosus, renal failure, hepatitis, and some malignancies will also have a *normochromic–normocytic anemia* of chronic inflammation where their RBC color and cell size will be normal but their hemoglobin will be low.

34. There are many drugs that can increase the risk of constipation especially with older adults, which include the following:

   A. Beta blockers and calcium channel blockers

   B. Opioids and diuretics

   C. NSAIDs and ACE inhibitors

   D. Dilantin and phenobarbital

35. Older adults have multiple comorbidities so they may have anemia of chronic disease. An example of this is when the RBC indices are within normal but the hemoglobin is low, which is caused by

   A. Chronic renal disease

   B. Myocardial infarction

   C. Glaucoma

   D. Diabetes mellitus type 2

36. Older adults who are diagnosed with the following leukemia generally have a chromosomal translocation, the Philadelphia chromosome.

   A. Acute myeloid leukemia

   B. Chronic myeloid leukemia

   C. Acute lymphocytic leukemia

   D. Chronic lymphocytic leukemia

37. The benchmark diagnostic screening test for vitamin D level is the

   A. Fat soluble vitamin screen profile

   B. Serum vitamin D level

   C. Serum 25(OH)D level

   D. Urine vitamin D level

38. The normal range for vitamin D is

   A. Less than 20 ng/ml

   B. More than 75 ng/ml

   C. Between 20 and 30 ng/ml

   D. More than 100 ng/ml

39. Paul Retire, 75 years old, has had osteoarthritis for several years. He has developed bony protuberances on his distal interphalangeal joints (DIPS) called

   A. Bouchard's nodules

   B. Murphy's tenderness points

   C. Heberden's nodes

   D. Ryan papules

40. Mr. Smith, 86 years old, presents with three "growths" which he says are relatively new. He complains of them "being like a wart, with a greasy texture, kind of like they are stuck on with glue" and on his neck and shoulders. Most likely they are

   A. Basal cell carcinoma

   B. Seborrheic keratoses

   C. Actinic keratosis

   D. Squamous cell carcinoma

6

Nurse Practitioner Role and Nurse–Patient Relationship

The Nurse Practitioner Role

The Gerontological Nurse Practitioner (GNP) role is autonomous but operates within the guidelines set by the regulations for each individual state. The role has greatly evolved from the inception of the first nurse practitioner (NP) role in the sixties. Prescriptive authority, either full or partial with a collaborating physician or under the direction of a physician, is granted to NPs certified to practice as GNPs in most states. Each state has its own State Nurse Practice Act and Board of Nursing that controls the scope of practice for NPs. The *Pearson Report, The Annual Legislative Update* is available at *http//:www.webnp.net*, which describes the NP's scope of practice in each state.

The American Nurses Association (ANA) describes an advanced practice nurse, such as a GNP, as a post baccalaureate educated nurse who is involved in practice. *The Nursing's Social Public Policy Statement and Nursing: Scope and Standards of Practice* (2004) specifically delineates the education, certification, and licensure for advanced practice nurses, which include NPs, clinical nurse specialists, nurse anesthetists, and nurse midwives.

The National Organization of Nurse Practitioner Faculties' (NONPF) most recent revision of competencies for the GNP role was in 2006 and is what all accredited graduate nursing programs follow in teaching educational curriculum for GNP students. Once the Consensus Model for APRN Regulation: Licensure, Accreditation, Certification, and Education of 2015 is implemented, there will be no more GNP role but rather a combined adult nurse practitioner (ANP)/GNP role. The competencies for this combined NP role have been developed for the primary care role, and the competencies for an acute role are being developed. The 2006 competencies, which are what the certification bodies are following until 2015, are accessible at *http://www.nonpf.com/associations/10789/files/DomainsandCoreComps2006.pdf*.

The competencies for the ANP/GNP role for primary care are accessible at *http://www.nonpf.com/displaycommon.cfm?an=1&subarticlenbr=30*. These competencies include being able to demonstrate competency in the NP role when managing and delivering care, being able to work collaboratively with all members of the interdisciplinary team, advocate for older adults on health policy issues, deliver safe and high quality care, and lead and mentor other health care professionals in the care of the older adult.

The Consensus Model for APRN Regulation (2008) is available at *http://www.nonpf.com/displaycommon.cfm?an=1&subarticlenbr=26* and standardizes the preparation, licensure, and maintenance of competency. This landmark document specifies titles for advanced practice nurses, delineates the specialties of advanced practice, and describes the new role with population foci for each of the six types of NP.

GNPs are able to work in a variety of health care delivery settings caring for older adults such as primary care, internal medicine, urgent care clinics, sub acute facilities, long-term care, visiting nurse agencies, assisted living agencies specialized for older adults, community health centers, palliative care, women's health, in the hospital on gerontology units, and a variety of entrepreneurial settings created specifically for older adults. Some GNPs are opening their own clinics especially in rural areas and running their business/practice independently depending on their State Nurse Practice Act. Other GNPs use teleconferencing to deliver care to older adults who have limited access to a provider.

The role of the NP has been studied to determine if NP patient outcomes are similar, less than, or better than that of physicians in primary care. The classic study conducted by Mundinger et al. (2000) found equal outcomes for physicians and NPs regarding health status, patient satisfaction, and physiological test results. A follow-up study of this randomized study in 2004 found equivalent outcomes by the NPs and the physicians (Lenz, Mundinger, Kane, Hopkins, & Lin, 2004). Other studies have generated similar results, and some (Laurant et al., 2006; Wilson et al., 2005) have found NP outcomes better than physicians.

The GNP role is influenced by reflective practice and is constantly expanding its role and scope of practice. It is patient centered versus disease focused like the physician's role. The GNP is involved in evidence-based practice and translational research, uses change management theory to expand on the NP scope of practice, applies theory from the liberal arts and sciences to critically think and analyze different options of care management, and is involved in inter- and intraprofessional collaboration and consultation.

The Nurse Practitioner–Patient Relationship

NPs develop respectful and collegial relationships with their older adult patients and often with their families. It behooves the GNP to work collaboratively with the older adult and family to develop a mutually agreed-upon plan of care and health regimen. The 2006 GNP Competencies that certification bodies are following until 2015 are accessible at *http://www.nonpf .com/associations/10789/files/DomainsandCoreComps2006.pdf* and list the following as areas for GNPs to discuss with older adult patients: suicidal prevention, potential for self-injury, sexually related issues, finances, risk taking behaviors they should avoid, possible substance abuse, independence, potential for abuse, and prognosis.

Family Involvement

The NP can be instrumental in providing respite support for family members caring for older adults. Caregiver burden includes the financial, social, psychological, and physical issues that a caregiver for an older adult relative or friend experiences. Organizing paid and/or volunteer staff to take over for the family members in caring for the older adult in the family is a very effective program that allows family to keep their elder home longer. In today's world, many households do not have anyone home to care and visit the older family members until the evening or even the weekends. Programs can be set up such as older adult day care, support seminars for caregivers to gain emotional support, volunteer programs to assist caregivers in caring for older adult family member, and design same-stop health care services frequently used by older adults to increase ease of family caring for their loved ones. Most people are inclined to say they would rather stay in their own home or with family than go into a nursing home. Having the above-mentioned services are imperative in a community to maximize the time and quality of family caregivers in keeping their older loved ones home as long as possible.

Many family members are not well equipped to manage the physical, psychosocial, and functional needs of an older adult with multiple end-stage chronic illnesses who need assistance with their activities of daily living. Caring for an older adult with multiple needs is burdensome for most people used to working full time and caring for their own children. Some families feel they cannot care for their loved older adults and need assistance in finding a suitable placement for their loved one or help in gaining home aids. GNPs can assist in providing the support and knowledge for caregivers. The newer assisted living facilities that allow as much independence as capable are an option that allows individuals to buy into the facility. So they can have independence and still have the choice to transfer to an area in the facility that provides more assistance such as light housekeeping and meals when the time comes. These programs also have an area for individuals who require total assistance. This progressive care type of facility is suitable for someone who wants to be as independent as possible but still have access to more services as one needs it.

Family care giving presents many problems when the person needing assistance has dementia or needs total help with activities of daily living. The GNP can assist the family in accessing the aging services such as Meals on Wheels and Senior Citizen Centers in the community that can assist the family in keeping their older loved one home. Caregivers need a phone number to reach someone to assist them in case of emergency since many of these emergencies will not be life threatening to the patient and demand a 911 call. Cahill, Lewis, Barg, and Bogner (2009) studied adults older than 65 years of age regarding their perception of having a family caregiver care for them when the time came. Results indicated the older adults did not want to impact their children's lives, felt guilty about being a burden to their family, and were worried that their children were overly anxious about their health. This reinforces the importance of having a family meeting and discussing all alternatives and trying to plan ahead for these care giving needs.

Teaching–Coaching

NPs often work with a physician(s) and are responsible for the majority of health teaching that occurs with patients and their families. In many instances providers, both physicians and NPs, serve as coach for both the patient and the family in transitioning to a nursing home, moving out of one's lifetime home, or other specific milestones that occur with older adults.

Some practices have little to no health teaching resources and likewise no handouts to give patients at their presentation for assistance on a specific issue. The GNP is in a unique position to develop brochures and handouts and offer seminars for family and/or older adults on a variety of issues using teaching/learning styles that are well received by older adults such as reviewing brochures, role modeling, discussion, demonstration and return demonstration, reinforcement of key principles, and review of the content presented. Being sure to use the correct language and level of literacy as well as the appropriate knowledge is paramount to successful health teaching. Additionally, setting up a comfortable learning environment that allows both older adults and their caregivers to gain the new knowledge at their own pace is necessary. Building the content from simple to complex and using examples to demonstrate key points can assist the NP in being successful in accomplishing the teaching goals. Giving suggestions for how to assess readiness to learn and motivate learners and assisting family members and the older adults in question as well as reinforcing the importance of compliance to health maintenance are all part of the GNP's role in health teaching. Strategies for communicating easily and effectively with home health aides and others who will assist the older adults with their activities of daily living should be discussed. In addition, a thorough explanation of the patient's community health resources should be given to the older adult and family.

The clinical UpToDate, evidence-based, and peer-reviewed resource can give many ideas for developing programs/in-services and handouts on a variety of health care issues written for providers, patients, educators, and institutions. This web-based resource is available for a limited fee at *http:// www.uptodate.com/home/index.html*. Other national guidelines for caring for patients with asthma (*http://www.nhlbi.nih.gov/guidelines/asthma*), hyperlipidemia (*http://www.theheart.org/article/148997.do.*), and diabetes (*http:// www.diabetes.org/formedia/2009/cpr-2010-a1c-diagnostic-tool.html*) have comprehensive management plans, illustrations, explanations of pathophysiology, checklists for patients and caregivers in documenting administration of medication and results, and effective strategies that have worked for others with similar disease states are all available at the respective Web sites. Suggestions for overcoming learning barriers for teaching are also available at these Web sites. The GNP can coach the family and older adult along the learning continuum as they become more comfortable with new living arrangements and roles in the family.

Health Literacy

The Institute of Medicine has described the problems people experience in understanding their health and treatment options as well as their access for health interventions (2004). For older adults, health literacy is compounded by variables such as not being able to see to read the directions of prescriptions and other health products, poor living arrangements far from services, not being able to drive or obtain a ride to health care offices, lack of funds, and multiple other problems that come with aging and many chronic illnesses. Health literacy for older adults is well described by the U.S. Department of Health and Human Services Web site, accessible at *http://www.health .gov/communication/literacy/olderadults/literacy.htm*. There is a review of health literacy, techniques for assisting older adults regarding communication, and exemplars of best practice for health literacy. The *Quick Guide to Health Literacy* is accessible at *www.health.gov/communication/literacy/ quickguide*. Healthy People 2020 includes health literacy improvement as one of its priority goals since the goal is to improve the health of populations and reduce disparities. A simple definition is given as follows: health literacy is about how the people understand what has been told them about their health and what they can choose to do with this information. The Healthy People 2020 document illustrates how health informatics technology, health literacy, and health communication can be addressed as a cohort so that more goals can be accomplished (*http://www.ncbi.nlm.nih .gov/bookshelf/br.fcgi?book=nap12474&part=ch5*). There are many literacy tasks the GNPs can assist their patients and families with, so their understanding is increased regarding the older adult's health situation including using information, analyzing abstract concepts, presenting information, calculating, and writing. GNPs must assist the older adults so they can become full, active partners in their health (Rajda & George, 2009). These same authors recommend that all older adults be screened for their health literacy by using *The REALM: Rapid Estimate of Adult Literacy in Medicine*, which is accessible through the Center for Health Care Strategies at *http://www.chcs .org/*, and always to assess the reading level of materials one gives out to patients and families.

Special Issues Impacting Older Adults for Nurse Practitioners

PALLIATIVE CARE

The End of Life Nursing Education Consortium (ELNEC), accessible at *www .aacn.nche.edu/ELNEC*, provides education and training for nurses regarding palliative care and end-of-life issues and suggests guidelines for use regarding pain and other symptom management for those individuals in late stages of their chronic illness and other terminal patients. Using an interdisciplinary approach, NPs can coordinate the health care team to maximize the quality of palliative care patients in long-term care as well as with the patient's family. There has been a trend to change from viewing the end-of-life or terminal care period of life to one of a palliative care approach for people who are in advanced stages of a disease. Quaglietti, Blum, and Ellis (2004) describe the following as the goal of palliative care: to prevent and assist with alleviating suffering while providing high quality of life for the patient/ family with a life-limiting disease. This is similar to the change in care focus to more of a biopsychosocial than a disease-management perspective (Fine & MacLow, 2004). The idea was to begin palliative care earlier in managing patients with advanced chronic disease so that patients were pain free and the management plan was more "care" than "cure" oriented. NPs can be reimbursed by Medicare for their care with patients as they go from palliative to terminal care.

Carter and Chichin (2003) suggest using the Minimum Data Set (MDS) as a tool to screen residents of long-term care facilities regarding their functional and health status to determine whether they are at high risk for deterioration and may benefit from palliative care. Fine and MacLow (2004) recommend the use of weight loss and change in ability to do activities of daily living independently as possible predictors of older adults who may warrant palliative care services.

ADVANCED DIRECTIVES

There is no doubt many deaths occur in long-term care facilities. In fact, the National Center for Health Statistics (2008) state approximately one in five deaths is in nursing homes. NPs and other providers have a responsibility to assist patients and their families in developing an advanced directive for the patient that addresses cardiopulmonary resuscitation, desire for hospitalization if condition deteriorates, nutrition, and use of antibiotics. It is suggested by Fine and MacLow (2004) that the GNP or physician discusses advanced directives with the family and patient upon admission to the long-term care facility so that the highest quality of life care can be given. People should have an advanced directive before they are old and acutely ill and GNPs can certainly recommend their patients to have one drawn up when they initially meet the patient in their practice setting. In order to have proof of an individual's wishes regarding their health care, it is important to have the following written documentation. A durable power of attorney for health is developed with an attorney to give a person the chance to designate a proxy to make decisions for them whether they should need assistance. Additionally, a living will is established to document the individual's wishes regarding his or her health if the need should arise. Advanced directives and goals of care should not be left unwritten since one does not know what acute health events may occur and be life threatening.

CULTURAL AWARENESS

NPs need to be able to provide quality care to diverse populations with varying cultural characteristics (JACHO, 2008). Weak cultural knowledge and lack of exposure to cultural diversity decreases ability to assess patients' cultural needs (Reeves & Fogg, 2006). Cultural humility is an ongoing process of self-awareness to identify different beliefs, values, and practices of people from different cultures. NPs can build relationships on similarities between themselves and others not differences. By not having personal biases and stereotyping individuals with specific ethnicities, religion, or views about euthanasia or environmental protection and so on, a GNP can be culturally aware and render high quality care. It is important for the NP to integrate the patient's values, health beliefs, and behaviors into the mutually planned care regimen and to be aware of how that individual's culture may impact their compliance. An example of a cultural assessment tool is Awareness, Skill, Knowledge, Encounters, and Desire (ASKED) developed by Campinha-Bacote (1999).

ELDER ABUSE/NEGLECT

Older adults are more likely to sustain serious injury from any physical abuse as compared to other people except for infants (Brown, Streubert, & Burgess, 2004). Approximately 10% of older adults are neglected or abused in the United States. Only one in fourteen elder abuse cases is reported (Muehlbauer & Crane, 2006). Given the increasing amount of individuals older than 65 years of age, there will likely be more and more elder abuse. Ninety percent of abusers of older adults are reported to be family members, but this is not likely to be accurate given the large number of older adults are not living with family at the end of their life (Fulmer, Guadagno, Bitondo-Dyer, & Connolly, 2004).

The health care provider is responsible for reporting any suspected abuse or neglect to the appropriate state protective agency. It behooves the GNP to document comprehensively any symptoms or signs of injury along with verbatim quotes from the individual even if abuse/neglect is not suspected at the time. Health care providers can distribute or put on their Web site or office bulletin boards copies of the local and state protective resources available. It is significant that GNPs be able to connect with abuse/neglect protective agencies easily so that appropriate screening may be done by investigative staff. The National Center on

Elder Abuse was developed as a clearinghouse of resources, which can be accessed at *http://www.ncea.aoa.gov/ncearoot/Main_Site/index.aspx.* Many times older adults are not totally honest about their injuries if they were abused by relatives since they consider themselves a burden and feel they have no other place to live but with their relatives. Abdominal assault that causes injury in older adults is often life threatening and leads to fatality five times more often than with other age groups (Brown et al., 2004). Other areas of physical abuse include genital injury from intimate partner abuse or rape and chest wall injury, which often involves hospitalization. Older adults are vulnerable for sexual abuse and the GNP will need to assess for this by asking specific questions related to any suspicious signs and symptoms. GNPs will need to be sensitive about asking their patients questions to maximize their safety at home or in any setting.

DRIVING

Many older adults continue to drive even into their nineties. Given the longer life span of individuals today, there is an increased number of older adults driving. Aging does not necessarily correlate with more driving accidents but rather an increased number of accidents may be because of having certain health conditions that impact reaction time, cognitive decision making, and visual dysfunction. There is a greater chance of fatality for older adults involved in motor vehicle accidents than with younger people (Margolis, Kerani, McGovern, Songer, Cauley, & Ensrud, 2002).

There are some older adults who know they should not be driving due to visual problems, cognitive changes, muscle weakness and tremors, cardiac dysrhythmias, seizure disorders, or from being on medications that may cloud their decision making or make them drowsy. These adults may need assistance in making the decision to quit driving, and the GNP is in a unique position to recommend that they find alternative transportation and that relinquishing their driving license is the "right thing to do" in order to maximize safety for all travelers on the roads. It is imperative that each older adult be assessed regarding the ability to keep driving. Certainly a mini-mental exam, sensory, musculoskeletal, cardiac, and neurologic exams as well as general appearance, affect, and level of thought processes should be comprehensively conducted. There are multiple sources of transportation and members of volunteer groups who drive older adults to health appointments, shopping, and recreation centers. Most states do not have any laws mandating an older adult be tested at certain ages, so it is generally up to the patient, family, and provider to assist the older adult regarding the decision of quitting driving.

HEALTH CARE DISPARITIES AMONG THE ELDERLY

All GNPs must be familiar with Healthy People 2010 and 2020 and follow the guidelines to assist with decreasing the gap in health care disparities among older adults. Through the development of new technology and greater emphasis on health promotion, people who are older than 65 number about one in every eight Americans, and it is projected there will be a 19% increase in the number of these older adults by 2030. In the year 2008, there were approximately 38.9 million people aged older than 65, representing approximately 12.8% of the total population (Administration on Aging, 2008). Black older adults comprise 8.3% of the older adult population or 3.2 million, and this group is expected to grow to 11% of the older population by 2050. As of 2008, there were 2.7 million Hispanic older individuals or 6.8% of the older adult population was older than 65 years, and this number is projected to increase by 17 million and comprise 19.8% of the older adult population by 2050. Therefore, it is predicted that by 2050, 32.6% or one-third of the older adult population will be Black and Hispanic. While older adults are healthier than they have been in the past, they tend to have both acute and chronic medical illnesses and are in need of health care. The percentage of older adults with chronic illnesses continues to increase, and their most frequently seen chronic conditions include hypertension, arthritis, cardiovascular disease, cancer, diabetes, and sinusitis (Administration on Aging, 2008). Eighty percent of older adults more than 65 years have one chronic disease and 50% have at least two comorbidities. It is crucial that GNPs are aware of the high risks that diverse older adults are especially susceptible and that they generally have more chronic illnesses than nondiverse older adults.

Conclusions

This chapter describes the role of the GNP and strategies for the GNP to use when dealing with multiple issues common to older adults. Caregiver needs, health literacy, health teaching, coaching the older adult and family, along with some specific issues that impact older adults such as cultural competency, elder abuse, driving, end-of-life and palliative care, and health care disparities among the elderly are discussed with relation to the GNP role. The GNP is in a unique position to advocate for the older adult and the family in establishing the best possible quality of life for the patient at home, in the hospital, or in a long-term care facility.

REFERENCES

Administration on Aging. (2008). *Minority aging.* Retrieved March 24, 2010, from http://www.aoa.gov/aoaroot/aging_statistics/minority_aging/Index.aspx

American Diabetes Association. (2009). *American Diabetes Association's new clinical practice recommendations promote A1C as diagnostic test for diabetes.* Retrieved May 6, 2010, from http://www.diabetes.org/for-media/2009/cpr-2010-a1c-diagnostic-tool.html

American Nurses Association. (2004). *Nursing: Scope and standards of practice.* Washington, DC: Author.

Brown, K., Streubert, G. E., & Burgess, A. W. (2004). Effectively detect and manage elder abuse. *The Nurse Practitioner, 29*(8), 22–31.

Cahill, E., Lewis, L., Barg, F., & Bogner, H. (2009). "You don't want to burden them": Older adults' views on family involvement in care. *Journal of Family Nursing, 15*(3), 295–317.

Campinha-Bacote, J. (1999). A model and instrument for addressing cultural competence in health care. *Journal of Nursing Education, 38,* 204.

Carter, J., & Chichin, E. (2003). Palliative care in the nursing home. In R. Morrison & D. Meir (Eds.), *Geriatric palliative care* (pp. 357–374). New York: Oxford University Press.

Center for Health Care Strategies. (2009). *The REALM: Rapid Estimate of Adult Literacy in Medicine.* Retrieved June 13, 2010, from http://www.chcs.org/

End of Life Nursing Education Consortium. (2010). *End of life care.* Retrieved May 22, 2010, from http://www.aacn.nche.edu/ELNEC

Fine, P., & MacLow, C. (2004). *Hospice referral and care: Practice guidance for clinicians.* Retrieved June 11, 2020, from http://cme.medscape.com/viewprogram/3345

Fulmer, T., Guadagno, L., Bitondo-Dyer, C., & Connolly, M. T. (2004). Progress in elder abuses screening and assessment instruments. *Journal of the American Geriatrics Society, 52,* 297–304.

Healthy People 2020. (2010). *Health literacy, e-health, and communication.* Retrieved June 13, 2010, from http://www.ncbi.nlm.nih.gov/bookshelf/br.fcgi?book=nap12474&part=ch5

Institute of Medicine. (2004). *Health literacy.* Retrieved May 22, 2010, from http://www.iom.edu/Activities/PublicHealth/RtblHealthLiteracy.aspx

Laurant, M., Reeves, D., Hermens, R., Braspenning, J., Grol, R., & Sibbald, B. (2006). Substitution of doctors by nurses in primary care. *Cochrane Database of Systematic Reviews,* (1).

Lenz, E., Mundinger, M., Kane, R., Hopkins, S., & Lin, S. (2004). Primary care outcomes in patients treated by nurse practitioners or physicians: Two-year follow-up. *Medical Care Research and Review, 61*(3), 332–351.

Margolis, K., Kerani, R., McGovern, P., Songer, T., Cauley, J., & Ensrud, K. (2002). Risk factors for motor vehicle crashes in older women. *The Journals of Gerontology, 57*(3), 186–191.

Muehlbauer, M., & Crane, P. (2006). Elder abuse and neglect. *Journal of Psychosocial Nursing, 44*(11), 43–48.

Mundinger, M., Kane, R., Lenz, E., Tsai,W-Y., Cleary, P., Friedewald, W., et al. (2000). Primary care outcomes in patients treated by nurse practitioners or physicians. *Journal of the American Medical Association. 283*(1), 59–69.

National Center on Elder Abuse: Administration on Aging. (2010). Retrieved June 4, 2010, from http://www.ncea.aoa.gov/ncearoot/Main_Site/index.aspx

National Cholesterol Education Program (NCEP)–Adult Treatment Panel (ATP) III Guidelines (2010). Retrieved March 23, 2010, from http://www.theheart.org/article/148997.do

National Health Statistics Report. (2008). *End of life care in nursing homes: Nursing home survey.* Retrieved June 5, 2010, from http://www.cdc.gov/nchs/data/nhsr/nhsr009.pdf

National Organization of Nurse Practitioner Faculties. (2006). *Domains and competencies for the gerontological nurse practitioner practice.* Retrieved June 6, 2010, from http://www.nonpf.com/associations/10789/files/DomainsandCore Comps2006.pdf

National Organization of Nurse Practitioner Faculties. (2008). *Consensus Model for APRN Regulation: Licensure, Accreditation, Certification, and Education.* Retrieved June 11, 2010, from http://www.nonpf.com/displaycommon. cfm?an=1&subarticlenbr=26

National Organization of Nurse Practitioner Faculties. (2010). *Domains and competencies for the Adult/Gero primary care NP practice.* Retrieved June 6, 2010, from http://www.nonpf.com/displaycommon.cfm?an=1&subarticlenbr=30

Quaglietti, S., Blum, L., & Ellis, V. (2004). The role of the adult health nurse practitioner in palliative care. *Journal of Hospice and Palliative Nursing, 6*(4), 209–214.

Rajda, C., & George, N. (2009). The effect of education and literacy levels on health outcomes of the elderly. *The Journal for Nurse Practitioners, 2,* 115–119.

Reeves, J., & Fogg, C. (2006). Perceptions of graduating nursing students regarding life experiences that promote culturally competent care. *Journal of Transcultural Nursing, 17,* 171–178.

The Joint Commission. (2008). *Hospitals, language, and culture.* Retrieved June 15, 2010, from http://www.jointcommission.org/PatientSafety/HLC/HLC_Develop_ Culturally_Competent_Pt_Centered_Stds.htm

United States Department of Health and Human Services. (2010). *The quick guide to health literacy.* Retrieved May 12, 2010, from www.health.gov/communication/literacy/quickguide

UpToDate. (2010). *Clinical resources for providers, educators, patients, or institutions.* Retrieved June 4, 2010, from http://www.uptodate.com/home/index.html.

Wilson, I., Landon, B., Hirschhorn, L., McInnes, K., Ding, L., Marsden, P., et al. (2005). Quality of HIV care provided by nurse practitioners, physician assistants, and physicians. *Annals of Internal Medicine, 143,* 729–736.

National Heart, Lung, & Blood Institute. (2010) *Guidelines for treatment of asthma.* Retrieved March 25, 2010, from http://www.nhlbi.nih.gov/guideines/asthma

TEST QUESTIONS

1. The following documentation and regulatory body controls the scope of practice for NPs in the United States:

   A. Nurse Practice Act and State Board of Nursing

   B. APRN certification and federal government

   C. American Nurses Association Scope of Practice for Advanced Practice Nurses and state government

   D. MSN masters degree and federal government

2. In 2015, The Consensus Model for Advanced Practice Nursing Regulation will be implemented. The four components of this model include

   A. Accreditation of BSN program, certification, DEA licensure, and APRN licensure

   B. Accreditation of MSN program, DEA licensure, Identification Pin, and competency simulation exam status

   C. Accreditation, licensure, education, and certification

   D. Certification, APRN licensure, DEA licensure, and Identification Pin

3. The term *caregiver burden* includes the following issues that a relative/friend caregiver assumes for an older adult who needs assistance with their care and activities of daily living:

   A. Social, religious, spiritual, and basic food and housing needs

   B. Basic food and housing needs, religious, psychosocial, and emotional needs

   C. Financial, spiritual, housing, and food requirements

   D. Financial, social, psychological, and physical needs

4. Teaching strategies that have shown success with older adults accomplishing the goals set up with the NP regarding their health include

   A. Demonstration and role modeling of the content

   B. Assigning an Internet reading and homework for the next care visit

   C. Financial incentive and pre-assigned reading for each care visit

   D. Ensuring a comfortable environment for teaching and giving a pre- and post-test of the content

5. The following document illustrates how health informatics technology, health literacy, and health communication can be addressed as a cohort so that more goals can be accomplished:

   A. Health Informatics for Older Adults

   B. Healthy People 2010/2020

   C. *Quick Guide to Health Literacy*

   D. *The REALM: Rapid Estimate of Adult Literacy in Medicine*

6. Research in long-term care indicates the following two predictors of older adults who may warrant palliative care services for their deteriorating end-stage chronic illness(es):

   A. Mental status and ability to take oral food

   B. Incontinence status and mental alertness state

   C. Weight loss and independent ability with activities of daily living

   D. Ability to take oral food and pain status

7. Advanced directives are extremely important for older adults who are experiencing life-threatening situations regarding their end-stage chronic illness. The individual must have the following to designate a proxy to make their health care decisions for them whether they should need assistance:

   A. Durable power of attorney

   B. Trust directed documentation

   C. Release from their family for assistance with decisions

   D. Estate planning

8. The rationale for each individual to have a living will is to

   A. Fairly distribute one's assets after death

   B. Document the individual's wishes regarding his or her health if the need should arise.

   C. Cite the rationale for one's desires for burial after death

   D. Direct the care provider in determining whether the patient's organs can be used for transplant

9. The GNP can best increase cultural competence by

    A. Gaining knowledge about various cultures with regard to who makes the health care decisions for family members and learning other values and beliefs held by different ethnicities

    B. Ensuring that all patients have equal access to health care by advocating for more community health centers in the state

    C. Volunteering with the AmeriCares Organization in the nearest city at least twice a year

    D. Listening to CDs to become familiar with several other languages

10. Research indicates that older adults have more severe complications from abuse and neglect than younger people do. One of the most frequent complications is

    A. Pneumonia

    B. Myocardial infarction

    C. Death

    D. Infection

11. There are multiple areas that an older adult needs routine assessments to ensure the individual is competent to continue driving. These areas would comprise

    A. Dermatological and neurological

    B. Cardiac and neurological

    C. Musculoskeletal and respiratory

    D. Immunological and inflammatory

12. In order to increase compliance by older adults regarding their lifestyle and health regimen such as sticking to a low salt, well-balanced diet and exercising at least five times a day, the GNP would be wise to

    A. Build in outcome evaluation such as weight and blood pressure

    B. Continue to increase the dietary restriction and weight loss program so the patient does not get bored with regimen

    C. Establish a relationship with one of the family of the older adults and teach them how to work harder with their loved one

    D. Add an incentive such as a decreased cost for their co-payment for visits with the GNP

13. One of the most helpful resources for health care providers to use for screening for neglect or abuse is the

   A. Ombudsman services of community

   B. Elder hostel group in local area

   C. Affirmative action group in town

   D. National Center on Elder Abuse

14. A realistic goal for NPs to deliver best practice health care is to become culturally

   A. Practical

   B. Patient

   C. Aware

   D. Tolerant

15. Part of the goal of every nurse practitioner–patient relationship with older adults will revolve around

   A. Establishing a mutually respectful relationship

   B. Developing boundaries so the patient will not need to ever contact the provider on weekends

   C. Knowing the patient's designated "person in case of emergency" so that all communication can go through this individual instead of the older adult

   D. Keeping the older adult realistic about their life expectancy so that they can plan accordingly

7

Health Care Systems and Policy

As the population of older adults continues to age, the need to develop effective health care policy to govern the care of this population is evident. Older adults approach their later years with a number of health care conditions that require management to promote quality of life. Health care management requires effective policy and reimbursement plans to ensure that older adults receive the best care in the most cost-effective manner. This chapter provides an overview of health policy that impacts older adults. Quality improvement efforts across environments of care, and the GNP's role in this effort are explored. The chapter concludes with a discussion of major reimbursement systems for older adults including the potential for a greater use of long-term care insurance in the future.

Health Care Delivery Systems

- As a result of the vast improvements in health care technology, health care costs increased 12% to 14% per year in the 1970s and have continued to increase annually.

- Although the health care delivery system has improved vastly over the past century, many of the currently available interventions to detect diseases early and treat diseases effectively are not accessible to older adults because:

  - Many older adults are uninsured

  - Insurance might not cover a necessary test, procedure, or treatment

  - Many older adults lack transportation to health care providers

  - Primary providers of geriatric care are not widely available.

HEALTH CARE POLICY

GNPs must be aware of the role of health care policy that impacts the care of older adults. The competencies for graduate-prepared nurses in this area focus on understanding governmental actions, institutional decision making, and organizational standards related to state and federal government law. GNPs may participate in the development of health care policy through patient advocacy efforts at the institutional, local, state, national and global levels. Examples of this would be giving testimony at a state hearing or representing patient needs at a hospital-based committee. GNPs may also assist in the implementation of policy by designing patient care services that meet policy requirements.

SAFETY AND INSTITUTE OF MEDICINE

The Institute of Medicine in conjunction with the Quality and Safety Education for Nurses (QSEN), project funded by the Robert Wood Johnson Foundation and led by Drs. Linda Cronenwett and Gwen Sherwood at the University of North Carolina, Chapel Hill, has put forth a number of competencies for graduate-prepared nurses in relation to safe NP practice. These six competencies, as well as the knowledge, skills, and attitudes necessary to fulfill these competencies are listed in Table 7.1.

QUALITY IMPROVEMENT

The GNP's role in quality improvement efforts expands across environments of care. Quality improvement serves to "assure the consumer of nursing of a specified degree of excellence through continuous measurement and evaluation" (Schmadl, 1979, p. 462). While nursing is intimately involved in quality improvement efforts, quality improvement is a system level effort that includes all departments within a health care organization. Nursing research, evidence-based practice, and quality improvement are closely linked in which implementation of best research evidence into practice promotes the highest quality care for patients and the best working environment for all GNPs.

Efforts to promote quality improvement in environments where GNPs' work stems as far back as Florence Nightingale who attempted to integrate findings from her own clinical care observations into nursing practice to improve the care of patients during the Crimean war. Today, quality improvement is an essential component of all care delivery systems. In fact, failure to adhere to quality improvement standards and practices may result in nonpayment for services. This was demonstrated most recently in 2008 when Medicare began to refuse to reimburse hospitals for care associated with preventable injuries such as patient falls and pressure ulcers.

TABLE 7.1

Quality and Safety for Nursing Education (QSEN) Core Competencies for Advanced Practice

Patient-Centered Care

Definition: Recognize the patient or designee as the source of control and full partner in providing compassionate and coordinated care based on respect for patient's preferences, values, and needs.

Knowledge	Skills	Attitudes
Analyze multiple dimensions of patient centered care: ■ patient/family/ community preferences and values ■ coordination and integration of care ■ information, communication, and education ■ physical comfort and emotional support ■ involvement of family and friends ■ transition and continuity Analyze how diverse cultural, ethnic, spiritual, and social backgrounds function as sources of patient, family, and community values Analyze social, political, economic, and historical dimensions of patient care processes and the implications for patient-centered care Integrate knowledge of psychological, spiritual, social, developmental, and physiological models of pain and suffering	Elicit patient values, preferences, and expressed needs as part of clinical interview, diagnosis, implementation of care plan, and evaluation of care Communicate patient values, preferences, and expressed needs to other members of health care team Provide patient-centered care with sensitivity, empathy, and respect for the diversity of human experience Ensure that the systems within which one practices support patient-centered care for individuals and groups whose values differ from the majority or one's own. Assess and treat pain and suffering in light of patient values, preferences, and expressed needs	Value seeing health care situations "through patients' eyes" Respect and encourage individual expression of patient values, preferences, and expressed needs Value the patient's expertise with own health and symptoms Honor learning opportunities with patients who represent all aspects of human diversity Seek to understand one's personally held attitudes about working with patients from different ethnic, cultural, and social backgrounds Willingly support patient-centered care for individuals and groups whose values differ from one's own Value cultural humility Seek to understand one's personally held values and beliefs about the management of pain or suffering

(Continued)

TABLE 7.1 (Continued)

Knowledge	Skills	Attitudes
Analyze ethical and legal implications of patient-centered care Describe the limits and boundaries of therapeutic patient-centered care	Respect the boundaries of therapeutic relationships Acknowledge the tension that may exist between patient preferences and organizational and professional responsibilities for ethical care Facilitate informed patient consent for care	Value shared decision making with empowered patients and families, even when conflicts occur
Analyze strategies that empower patients or families in all aspects of the health care process	Engage patients or designated surrogates in active partnerships along the health—illness continuum	Respect patient preferences for degree of active engagement in care process
Analyze features of physical facilities that support or pose barriers to patient-centered care Analyze reasons for common barriers to active involvement of patients and families in their own health care processes	Create or change organizational cultures so that patient and family preferences are assessed and supported Assess level of patient's decisional conflict and provide access to resources Eliminate barriers to presence of families and other designated surrogates based on patient preferences	Honor active partnerships with patients or designated surrogates in planning, implementation, and evaluation of care Respect patient's right to access to personal health records Value system changes that support patient-centered care
Integrate principles of effective communication with knowledge of quality and safety competencies Analyze principles of consensus building and conflict resolution Analyze advanced practice nursing roles in assuring coordination, integration, and continuity of care Describe process of reflective practice	Continuously analyze and improve own level of communication skill in encounters with patients, families, and teams Provide leadership in building consensus or resolving conflict in the context of patient care Communicate care provided and needed at each transition in care Incorporate reflective practices into own repertoire	Value continuous improvement of own communication and conflict resolution skills Value consensus Value the process of reflective practice

(Continued)

Teamwork and Collaboration

Definition: Function effectively within nursing and inter-professional teams, fostering open communication, mutual respect, and shared decision making to achieve quality patient care.

Knowledge	Skills	Attitudes
Analyze own strengths, limitations, and values as a member of a team Analyze impact of own advanced practice role and its contributions to team functioning	Demonstrate awareness of own strengths and limitations as a team member Continuously plan for improvement in use of self in effective team development and functioning Act with integrity, consistency, and respect for differing views	Acknowledge own contributions to effective or ineffective team functioning
Describe scopes of practice and roles of all health care team members Analyze strategies for identifying and managing overlaps in team member roles and accountabilities	Function competently within own scope of practice as a member of the health care team Assume role of team member or leader based on the situation Guide the team in managing areas of overlap in team member functioning Solicit input from other team members to improve individual, as well as team, performance Empower contributions of others who play a role in helping patients/families achieve health goals	Respect the unique attributes that members bring to a team, including variation in professional orientations, competencies, and accountabilities Respect the centrality of the patient/family as core members of any health care team
Analyze strategies that influence the ability to initiate and sustain effective partnerships with members of nursing and inter-professional teams Analyze impact of cultural diversity on team functioning	Initiate and sustain effective health care teams Communicate with team members, adapting own style of communicating to needs of the team and situation	Appreciate importance of inter-professional collaboration Value collaboration with nurses and other members of the nursing team

(Continued)

TABLE 7.1 (Continued)

Knowledge	Skills	Attitudes
Analyze differences in communication style preferences among patients and families, advanced practice nurses, and other members of the health care team	Communicate respect for team member competence in communication Initiate actions to resolve conflict	Value different styles of communication
Describe impact of own communication style on others		
Describe examples of the impact of team functioning on safety and quality of care Analyze authority gradients and their influence on teamwork and patient safety	Follow communication practices that minimize risks associated with handoffs among providers and across transitions in care Choose communication styles that diminish the risks associated with authority gradients among team members Assert own position/perspective and supporting evidence in discussions about patient care	Appreciate the risks associated with handoffs among providers and across transitions in care Value the solutions obtained through systematic, inter-professional collaborative efforts
Identify system barriers and facilitators of effective team functioning Examine strategies for improving systems to support team functioning	Lead or participate in the design and implementation of systems that support effective teamwork Engage in state and national policy initiatives aimed at improving teamwork and collaboration	Value the influence of system solutions in achieving team functioning

Evidence-Based Practice (EBP)

Definition: Integrate best current evidence with clinical expertise and patient/family preferences and values for delivery of optimal health care.

Knowledge	Skills	Attitudes
Demonstrate knowledge of health research methods and processes	Use health research methods and processes, alone or in partnership with scientists, to generate new knowledge for practice	Appreciate strengths and weaknesses of scientific bases for practice

(Continued)

Describe evidence-based practice to include the components of research evidence, clinical expertise, and patient/family values	Adhere to Institutional Review Board guidelines Role model clinical decision making based on evidence, clinical expertise, and patient/family preferences and values	Value the need for ethical conduct of research and quality improvement Value all components of evidence-based practice
Identify efficient and effective search strategies to locate reliable sources of evidence	Employ efficient and effective search strategies to answer focused clinical questions	Value development of search skills for locating evidence for best practice
Identify principles that comprise the critical appraisal of research evidence	Critically appraise original research and evidence summaries related to area of practice	Value knowing the evidence base for practice specialty
Summarize current evidence regarding major diagnostic and treatment actions within the practice specialty	Exhibit contemporary knowledge of best evidence related to practice specialty	Value public policies that support evidence-based practice
Determine evidence gaps within the practice specialty	Promote research agenda for evidence that is needed in practice specialty	
	Initiate changes in approaches to care when new evidence warrants evaluation of other options for improving outcomes or decreasing adverse events	
Analyze how the strength of available evidence influences the provision of care (assessment, diagnosis, treatment, and evaluation)	Develop guidelines for clinical decision making regarding departure from established protocols/standards of care	Acknowledge own limitations in knowledge and clinical expertise before determining when to deviate from evidence-based best practices
Evaluate organizational cultures and structures that promote evidence-based practice	Participate in designing systems that support evidence-based practice	Value the need for continuous improvement in clinical practice based on new knowledge

(Continued)

TABLE 7.1 *(Continued)*

Quality Improvement (QI)

Definition: Use data to monitor the outcomes of care processes, and use improvement methods to design and test changes to improve continuously the quality and safety of health care systems.

Knowledge	Skills	Attitudes
Describe strategies for improving outcomes of care in the setting in which one is engaged in clinical practice	Use a variety of sources of information to review outcomes of care and identify potential areas for improvement	Appreciate that continuous quality improvement is an essential part of the daily work of all health professionals
Analyze the impact of context (such as access, cost, or team functioning) on improvement efforts	Propose appropriate aims for quality improvement efforts	
	Assert leadership in shaping the dialogue about and providing leadership for the introduction of best practices	
Analyze ethical issues associated with quality improvement	Assure ethical oversight of quality improvement projects	Value the need for ethical conduct of quality improvement
Describe features of quality improvement projects that overlap sufficiently with research, thereby requiring IRB oversight	Maintain confidentiality of any patient information used to determine outcomes of quality improvement efforts	
Describe the benefits and limitations of quality improvement data sources, and measurement and data analysis strategies	Design and use databases as sources of information for improving patient care	Appreciate the importance of data that allows one to estimate the quality of local care
	Select and use relevant benchmarks	
Explain common causes of variation in outcomes of care in the practice specialty	Select and use tools (such as control charts and run charts) that are helpful for understanding variation	Appreciate how unwanted variation affects outcomes of care processes
	Identify gaps between local and best practice	

(Continued)

Describe common quality measures in the practice specialty	Use findings from root cause analyses to design and implement system improvements	Value measurement and its role in good patient care
	Select and use quality measures to understand performance	
Analyze the differences between micro-system and macro-system change	Use principles of change management to implement and evaluate care processes at the micro-system level	Appreciate the value of what individuals and teams can to do to improve care
Understand principles of change management	Design, implement, and evaluate tests of change in daily work (using an experiential learning method such as Plan-Do-Study-Act)	Value local systems improvement (in individual practice, team practice on a unit, or in the macro-system) and its role in professional job satisfaction
Analyze the strengths and limitations of common quality improvement methods	Align the aims, measures, and changes involved in improving care	Appreciate that all improvement is change but not all change is improvement
	Use measures to evaluate the effect of change	

Safety

Definition: Minimizes risk of harm to patients and providers through both system effectiveness and individual performance.

Knowledge	Skills	Attitudes
Describe human factors and other basic safety design principles as well as commonly used unsafe practices (such as work-arounds and dangerous abbreviations)	Participate as a team member to design, promote, and model effective use of technology and standardized practices that support safety and quality	Value the contributions of standardization and reliability to safety
		Appreciate the importance of being a safety mentor and role model
Describe the benefits and limitations of selected safety-enhancing technologies (such as barcodes, Computer Provider Order Entry, and electronic prescribing)	Participate as a team member to design, promote, and model effective use of strategies to reduce risk of harm to self and others	Appreciate the cognitive and physical limits of human performance

(Continued)

TABLE 7.1 (Continued)

Knowledge	Skills	Attitudes
Evaluate effective strategies to reduce reliance on memory	Promote a practice culture conducive to highly reliable processes built on human factors research	
	Use appropriate strategies to reduce reliance on memory (such as forcing functions and checklists)	
Delineate general categories of errors and hazards in care Identify best practices for organizational responses to error Describe factors that create a just culture and culture of safety Describe best practices that promote patient and provider safety in the practice specialty	Communicate observations or concerns related to hazards and errors to patients, families, and the health care team Identify and correct system failures and hazards in care Design and implement micro-system changes in response to identified hazards and errors Engage in a systems focus rather than blaming individuals when errors or near misses occur Report errors and support members of the health care team to be forthcoming about errors and near misses	Value own role in reporting and preventing errors Value systems approaches to improving patient safety in lieu of blaming individuals Value the use of organizational error reporting systems
Describe processes used to analyze causes of error and allocation of responsibility and accountability (such as root cause analysis and failure mode effects analysis)	Participate appropriately in analyzing errors and designing, implementing, and evaluating system improvements	Value vigilance and monitoring of care, including one's own performance, by patients, families, and other members of the health care team
Describe methods of identifying and preventing verbal, physical, and psychological harm to patients and staff	Prevent escalation of conflict Respond appropriately to aggressive behavior	Value prevention of assaults and loss of dignity for patients, staff, and aggressors

(Continued)

| Analyze potential and actual impact of national patient safety resources, initiatives, and regulations | Use national patient safety resources:

■ for own professional development

■ to focus attention on safety in care settings

■ to design and implement improvements in practice | Value relationship between national patient safety campaigns and implementation in local practices and practice settings |

Informatics

Definition: Use information and technology to communicate, manage knowledge, mitigate error, and support decision making.

Knowledge	Skills	Attitudes
Contrast benefits and limitations of common information technology strategies used in the delivery of patient care Evaluate the strengths and weaknesses of information systems used in patient care	Participate in the selection, design, implementation, and evaluation of information systems Communicate the integral role of information technology in nurses' work Model behaviors that support implementation and appropriate use of electronic health records Assist team members to adopt information technology by piloting and evaluating proposed technologies	Value the use of information and communication technologies in patient care
Formulate essential information that must be available in a common database to support patient care in the practice specialty Evaluate benefits and limitations of different communication technologies and their impact on safety and quality	Promote access to patient care information for all professionals who provide care to patients Serve as a resource for how to document nursing care at basic and advanced levels	Appreciate the need for consensus and collaboration in developing systems to manage information for patient care

(Continued)

TABLE 7.1 (Continued)

Knowledge	Skills	Attitudes
	Develop safeguards for protected health information	Value the confidentiality and security of all patient records
	Champion communication technologies that support clinical decision making, error prevention, care coordination, and protection of patient privacy	
Describe and critique taxonomic and terminology systems used in national efforts to enhance interoperability of information systems and knowledge management systems	Access and evaluate high quality electronic sources of health care information	Value the importance of standardized terminologies in conducting searches for patient information
	Participate in the design of clinical decision-making supports and alerts	Appreciate the contribution of technological alert systems
	Search, retrieve, and manage data to make decisions using information and knowledge management systems	Appreciate the time, effort, and skill required for computers, databases, and other technologies to become reliable and effective tools for patient care
	Anticipate unintended consequences of new technology	

Reprinted with permission from Quality & Safety Education for Nurses. Competency KSAs (Graduate). (N.D.) Retrieved June 22, 2010 from *http://www.qsen.org/ksas_graduate.php*

Quality of care is a necessary element of quality improvement and is measured in a number of ways. Many health care agencies in which GNPs work have dedicated quality improvement teams who have implemented measurement practices in order to collect data to assure quality in the respective facilities. Examples of quality improvement measurements include, but are not limited to, the following:

■ Chart audits

■ Post-discharge patient interviews or surveys

■ Staff interviews/surveys

As described in the definition, quality improvement efforts are ongoing and continuous. Some have described quality improvement efforts in a linear direction toward quality. However, most authors describe quality improvement programs in a circular pattern, beginning with identification of the standard of care and moving toward the measurement of quality, promotion of actions toward quality and revisions to improve both the care and standards. Regardless of the model used by a given facility, measurement efforts directed toward quality usually result in the need to improve or maintain nursing practice.

The GNP plays an important role in quality improvement across environments of care. The role of the GNP is especially important when it comes to identification of standards and taking action to improve care. GNPs are change agents who are able to work with quality improvement teams to articulate a problem, review the current literature on a topic area, and select the best evidence and implement it into clinical practice. In fact, the more closely involved the GNP and nursing staff are with the quality improvement efforts in a system, the greater likelihood of success of these efforts. Sale (1996) reports that "Quality of care is the responsibility of everyone involved in health care and it was never more important than it is today" (p. 39).

One important way in which GNPs will work toward quality improvement in their health care environment is in helping to select standards of care. Standards of care are put forth by a variety of organizations to help guide institutions toward quality health care. Examples of organizations that produce documents related to scope and standards of health care practice include the following:

- State Departments of Health

- National Gerontological Nurse Association

- American Nurse Association

- National League for Nursing

- Specialty Nursing Organizations (such as Oncology Nurse Society)

- Joint Commission on Accreditation of Hospitals and Health Care Facilities.

In systems where quality improvement practices are designed and managed by a team, the GNP will also work with nursing staff members to ensure that documentation is effective in order to collect data to evaluate the outcomes of quality improvement efforts. The GNP may participate in quality improvement committees and possesses the expertise to facilitate evidence-based practice integration across environments of care. Selection of measurement tools for quality improvement and data collection may also involve the GNP.

Reimbursement

Reimbursement for health care has changed as a result of increasing costs. Allowable expenses under Medicare and Medicaid plans as well as private insurances have diminished in many cases and have been removed altogether in some cases. The lack of reimbursement for medications and treatments for illness and the inability to pay out of pocket for these expensive treatments have resulted in an increase in the rates of noncompliance or nonadherence to medication regimes. About half of all patients take the medications as prescribed upon leaving the physician's office. The other half take the medications incorrectly or not at all. One-third of those who take the medications incorrectly do not take them at all; one-third takes some of the medications prescribed; and one-third does not even fill the prescription.

Little, if any, time is spent on how to assist patients without health insurance to obtain needed health care. Regardless of the reason, many older adults need financial assistance to pay for health care. Often hospitals have programs to help older adults finance their health care over a period of months or to excuse the older adult from paying, if legitimately he or she cannot afford to do so. Physicians and other health care providers may offer the same payment alternatives for services received at private physicians' offices. Physicians in private practice may also have samples of medications to distribute to low-income older adults. Clinics often have sliding scales to make health care in these facilities more affordable. There are also various state-run programs that help older adults with resources for financing or finding health care that is affordable.

Older Americans Act

- Title III of the Older American's Act of 1965 directed attention toward public and private health care systems to provide improved access to services and advocacy for older adults.

- This program improved community services such as home-delivered meals, transportation, home health care and homemaking assistance, adult day care, home repair, and legal assistance—all of which allow many older adults to remain functionally independent and community dwelling.

- These programs are administered within local area agencies on aging (AAAs) in each state. AAAs provide older adults and health care providers with a resource to access and afford health care.

- To locate the AAA in each state, use the links tab located at *http://www .n4a.org*. In addition to this Web resource, the administration on aging offers a toll-free Eldercare Locator telephone number—(800) 677-1116—to help older adults, families, and health care providers obtain necessary community services throughout the United States. Operators at Eldercare Locator assist callers to find information and assistance to address health care and other issues to ensure high functioning and quality of life.

- In addition to AAAs, senior service offices in hospitals are good sources of information about hospital and community-based resources.

Medicare and Medigap

- Medicare is a federal program that was enacted into law in 1965 during a time in U.S. history known as The Great Society. Medicare was among several programs that were started during this period with the specific aim of assisting the poor, the disabled, and older people to have a better quality of health care and quality of life.

- Older adults who have not paid into the U.S. Social Security system, either because they were never employed or because they immigrated to the U.S. as older adults, must buy into the Medicare system to receive these benefits.

- The large majority of people aged 65 and older are enrolled in Medicare.

- To be eligible to receive Medicare, older adults must have contributed to Social Security or the Medicare system during their working years or had a spouse who had worked and contributed to these systems.

- Medicare is paid for by the government and therefore involves regulation, including the need for institutions receiving Medicare reimbursement to complete full resident assessment instruments within 14 days and a plan of care within 21 days of facility admission.

- Health care delivery under Medicare is provided by private physicians, hospitals, nurses, nurse practitioners, and various health care facilities, but not Medicare employees.

■ Private physicians who treat Medicare patients receive 80% of the usual customary and reasonable (UCR) fee for services provided if they accept Medicare assignment. If they do not, they can charge no more than 115% of the amount allowed by Medicare, and the client must pay the 20% remaining UCR and any other amount up to 115%.

■ Physicians are often hesitant to accept the low reimbursement for older adults through Medicare, and patients are hesitant to receive care from physicians who do not accept Medicare assignment because of the need to finance the co-pay. Consequently, there is a shortage of primary care physicians to treat the increasing health care needs of older adults.

■ Medicare has several parts.

■ Part A provides hospital insurance for older adults. In the event that an older adult requires hospitalization, this is the type of Medicare insurance that would pay for the hospital stay. In addition, this is the portion of Medicare that pays for short-term nursing home or home care visits after hospitalization for the older adult to return to prehospitalization health status. Medicare Part A also pays for hospice care (which is discussed in Chapter 7). Generally, there is no premium for this insurance. In other words, if older adults meet the eligibility for Medicare as stated previously, they are automatically enrolled in the Part A Medicare plan.

■ Part B pays for visits to physicians, nurse practitioners, and for other health care expenditures, such as x-rays, physical and occupational outpatient therapy, and laboratory tests. There is a monthly premium that older adults must pay for this type of Medicare plan. The current monthly premium is about $78. The amount is usually deducted from the recipient's monthly Social Security checks. Part B Medicare also requires recipients to pay the first $110 of charges before it will begin reimbursement. This is known as a deductible. The deductible for Part B Medicare is likely to increase annually. Coverage of Medicare for health care needs of older adults is detailed in Table 7.2.

■ Part C is the blending of both Medicare Part A and B but is administered through private insurance companies that have been approved by Medicare to manage the benefit.

■ Part D is the prescription drug coverage insurance that has been most recently added to Medicare. Many plans are available and most have a cost.

■ The Medicare traditional plan aforementioned has undergone much scrutiny since its inception in 1965. From a government perspective, providing Medicare coverage to an increasingly larger cohort of older adults is

TABLE 7.2

Medicare Coverage Guidelines

Service or Item	What Medicare Covers
Ambulance Services	Ambulance services when it is medically necessary for you to be transported to a hospital or skilled nursing facility, and transportation in any other vehicle would endanger your health. Medicare pays for ambulance transport to the nearest hospital or skilled nursing facility that provides the services you need.
Chiropractic Services	Manipulation of the spine to correct a subluxation (when one or more of the bones of your spine moved out of position).
Clinical Trials	Routine costs if you take part in a qualifying clinical trial. Clinical trials test new types of medical care, like how well a new cancer drug works. Clinical trials help doctors and researchers see whether the new care works and whether it is safe. It is important for you to ask what costs you will have to pay before signing up for a clinical trial. Note: Medicare does not cover the cost of experimental care, such as the drugs or devices being tested in a clinical trial.
Dental Services	Medicare does not cover routine dental care or most dental procedures such as cleanings, fillings, tooth extractions, or dentures. In rare cases, Medicare Part B will pay for certain dental services. In addition, Medicare Part A may pay for certain hospital stays for severe or complicated dental procedures, even when the dental care itself is not covered. Some Medicare Advantage Plans may offer additional dental coverage.
Diabetic Supplies	Medicare covers glucose testing monitors, blood glucose test strips, lancet devices and lancets, glucose control solutions, and therapeutic shows (in some cases). There may be limits on supplies or how often you get them. You should ask if the pharmacy or supplier is enrolled in the Medicare program. Note: Syringes and insulin (unless used with an insulin pump) are not covered.
Durable Medical Equipment	Items such as oxygen, wheelchairs, walkers, and hospital beds needed for use in the home.

(Continued)

TABLE 7.2 (Continued)

Service or Item	What Medicare Covers
Emergency Room Services (A medical emergency is when you believe that your health is in serious danger—when every second counts. You may have a bad injury, sudden illness, or an illness quickly getting much worse.)	Medicare covers emergency room services.
Eyeglasses	One pair of eyeglasses with standard frames that include an intraocular lens after cataract surgery.
Foot Exams	These exams are covered if you have diabetes-related nerve damage and meet certain conditions.
Hearing and Balance Exams	These exams are covered if your doctor orders them to see if medical treatment is needed. Routine screening exams are not covered.
Kidney Dialysis Services	Kidney dialysis with services and supplies, either in a facility or at home.
Long-term Care	Most long-term care, in a nursing home or at home, is custodial care (help with activities of daily living such as bathing, dressing, using the bathroom, and eating). Medicare does not cover long-term care, since it cannot cover custodial care when that is the only kind of care you need. Medicare Part A only covers skilled care given in a certified skilled nursing facility or in your home. You must meet certain conditions for Medicare to pay for skilled care when you get of the hospital.
Medical Nutrition Therapy Services	These services are covered for people who have diabetes or kidney disease (unless you are on dialysis) with a doctor's referral. Medical nutrition therapy services are covered for 3 years after a kidney transplant.

(Continued)

Mental Health Care	Medicare Part A covers impatient mental health care, including room, meals nursing, and other related services and supplies. Medical Part B covers mental health services generally given outside a hospital, including visits with a doctor clinical psychologist, or clinical social worker, and lab tests. Medicare Part B also covers partial hospitalization services for people who need intensive coordinated outpatient care to help them avoid impatient treatment.
Practitioner Services	Services provided by clinical social workers, physician assistants, and nurse practitioners.
Prescription Drugs	Except in a few cases (like certain cancer drugs), the Original Medicare Plan does not cover outpatient prescription drugs. If you are eligible to get drugs that are covered, you should ask whether the pharmacy is enrolled in the Medicare program. If the pharmacy is not enrolled, Medicare will not pay. Note: Medicare's new prescription drug coverage will start on January 1, 2006. Medicare-approved drug discount cards are available now.
Prosthetic/Orthotic Items	■ Arm, leg, back, and neck braces ■ Artificial eyes ■ Artificial limbs (and their replacement parts) ■ Breast prostheses (after mastectomy) ■ Prosthetic devices needed to replace an internal body part or function (including ostoncy supplies) Note: These items are considered durable medical equipment.
Second Surgical Opinions	Second surgical opinion by a doctor (in some cases). Sometimes, a third opinion may be covered.
Surgical Dressing	Dressings required for the treatment of a wound.
Telemedicine	Services in some rural areas.
Tests	X-rays, MRIs, CT scans, EKGs, and some other diagnostic tests if medically necessary.

(Continued)

TABLE 7.2 (Continued)

Service or Item	What Medicare Covers
Transplant Services	Heart, lung, kidney, pancreas, intestine, and liver transplants (under certain conditions and in Medicare-certified facilities only), and bone marrow and cornea transplants (under certain conditions). Oral immunosuppressive drugs if the transplant was paid for by Medicine, or paid by an employer group health plan that was required to pay before Medicare. You must have been entitled to Part A at the time of the transplant and entitled to Part B at the time you get immunosuppressive drugs, and the transplant must have been performed in a Medicare-certified facility.
Travel (outside the United States)	Except for some emergency services in Mexico and Canada, the original Medicare Plan does not cover health cure when you travel outside the United States. Some Medicare Advantage Plans, Medigap policies, and the Railroad Retirement Board have different rules. Check your insurance coverage before you travel outside the United States.
Urgently Needed Care (care you need for sudden illness or injury that is not a medical emergency)	Medicare Part B covers urgently needed care.

challenging and has resulted in limited reimbursement. Attempts to resolve some of these issues, numerous changes, and additions to the traditional Medicare plan have evolved.

- Medigap is private (nongovernmental) health insurance available to Medicare recipients for purchase to help pay for what Medicare does not cover.

  - Some of the health care expenses covered by Medigap include Medicare deductibles, co-pays (the additional amount of money that the patient must pay the health care provider), health care outside the United States, and medications.

  - The federal government has set regulations that must be followed by the providers of these plans.

  - There are 10 standard plans that must cover some of the essentials such as deductibles. However, each Medigap plan may also have additional benefits and set its own premiums.

- Many traditional Medicare recipients purchase a Medigap policy. However, some older Medicare patients cannot afford the monthly premiums for these supplemental plans.

- The Medicare Prescription Drug Improvement and Modernization Act of 2003 approved prescription discount drug cards for Medicare recipients. These cards are available to over 7 million of Medicare's 41 million participants. To be eligible for the discount cards, older adults must apply, and, depending on their income, a fee of $30 may be charged. The cards provide discounts on some, but not all, medications.

- Culture impacts health care reimbursement in which many older adults who have immigrated to the United States live their later lives with their adult children. Those who have not paid into the U.S. Social Security system must either buy into the Medicare system (the traditional health reimbursement program for older adults) or become eligible for Medicaid. However, legislation passed in the 1990s made it more difficult for older adults who were not U.S. citizens to access Medicaid, with the result that older adults may not have any way to pay for health care.

Medicare Managed Care, Prospective Payment Systems, and Other Medicare Systems

- Medicare Managed Care began a strong movement in the early 1990s in an attempt to lower the administrative costs associated with Medicare.

- Medicare recipients were asked to voluntarily select a health maintenance organization (HMO) to receive their health care.

- Health care received through these HMOs would be paid for by Medicare.

- Unfortunately, for the HMOs, older adults used considerably more health care services than Medicare reimbursed the HMO.

- Consequently, HMOs lost money, and, by 2000, many had withdrawn from the Medicare Managed Care business. While some HMOs still serve older adults in many parts of the country, many HMOs no longer take older adult Medicare clients.

- Because of the increasing cost of health care in the 1970s and 1980s, federal legislation in 1983 implemented a prospective payment system (PPS) that involved a set payment amount before care based on the diagnosis of the patient.

- This PPS was based on defined diagnostic related groups (Sultz & Young, 1999). This system set a limit on the amount of money the hospital would be reimbursed for hospital stays.

- As a result of the implementation of the PPS system, older adults tend to receive more surgery and other treatments on an outpatient basis.

- While there are certainly positive aspects of this change in health care delivery—such as the ability to meet health care goals more effectively at home and the ability to remain free from the risks of hospitalization—should a problem arise, the need to transport to a facility with appropriate resources may be necessary, and the delay in accessing these services could increase both morbidity and mortality.

- In further attempts to repair the problems in the Medicare system, three newer alternatives have evolved:

  - Preferred provider organizations provide discounts to older adults who choose primary care providers and specialists who have agreed to accept Medicare assignment for patients.

  - Medicare fee-for-service plans contract with private providers to allow older adults to go to any Medicare-approved doctor or hospital that is willing to take them. Benefits of these plans are improved coverage, such as extra hospital days. However, providers must work with private insurance plans directly to determine coverage for the health care expenditures. Moreover, an additional premium may be involved.

  - Specialty plans to meet the diverse and comprehensive needs of older adults are currently being developed. More information on these plans will be available as they become more widely utilized among older adults.

Medicaid

- Medicaid, a combined federal and state payment system, varies from state to state, but it funds health care, including nursing home care, for low-income older adults.

- Medicaid is a governmental program aimed at improving access to health care for indigent individuals.

- Medicaid is a state-administered welfare program of health care for all ages. In fact, half of Medicaid recipients are children.

- To be eligible for Medicaid, older adults must meet specific income and asset guidelines put forth by their state.

- Older people who have minimal financial resources and who qualify for income assistance through a federal program called Supplemental Security Income (SSI) also become eligible for Medicaid health care benefits.

- Persons aged 65 and older may have Medicare benefits and qualify for Medicaid.

- For older adults with limited assets and income, Medicaid may supplement Medicare benefits and pay for health care expenses not covered by Medicare, including medications, additional hospital or nursing home days, and durable medical equipment.

- For older adults who have both Medicare and Medicaid coverage for health care, Medicare is the primary payment system and Medicaid is secondary.

- The Centers for Medicare and Medicaid Services (2005) reports that Medicaid is currently the largest source of funding for health-related services for the poor in the United States.

- Medicaid was enacted by the same legislation as Medicare in 1965, also known as Title XIX of the Social Security Act.

- There is wide variability in covered medical expenses throughout the country.

- Each state establishes eligibility guidelines, allowable expenses, how much will be paid for these expenses, and how the program will be run within the state. Thus, there are as many different Medicaid programs as there are states. Mandated covered expenses for older adults include the following:

  - Inpatient and outpatient hospital services

  - Physician services

  - Nursing home services

  - Home care services that are delivered to prevent nursing home stays

  - Laboratory and x-ray services

- Many state Medicaid programs provide extended coverage for home- and community-based services if these services are keeping the older adult out of a covered nursing home stay that fall within a newer Medicaid program known as All-inclusive Care for the Elderly.

- The Personal Responsibility and Work Opportunity Reconciliation Act of 1996 welfare reform bill made legal resident aliens and other qualified aliens who entered the United States on or after that period ineligible for Medicaid for 5 years.

■ If an older adult is a Medicaid recipient, payment for health care expenses is provided directly to the health care provider.

■ Although Medicaid is used by all population groups in each state, the highest expenditures are made on behalf of older adults. While children average approximately $1,200 a year in Medicaid expenditure, older adults, who make up 9% of Medicaid recipients, average approximately $11,000 per person in annual Medicaid expenditures.

■ Medicaid payments for long-term care services utilized primarily by older adults were approximately $37.2 billion in 2001 (Centers for Medicare & Medicaid Services, 2005).

■ Medicaid has more enhanced coverage and fewer limitations than Medicare.

Long-Term Care Insurance

■ Long-term care insurance is a relatively new concept designed to meet the needs of the growing elderly population. It is likely that the role of long-term care insurance will expand greatly once health care is reformed.

■ The likelihood of older adults requiring long-term care at some point in time in their lives is approximately 50% (Alexander, 2005).

■ With an average stay of 19 months and an average cost of $30,000 per year, older adults cannot afford to pay out of pocket for nursing home stays.

■ Consequently, an illness that results in a nursing home stay has the potential to bankrupt most middle-income older adults.

■ Long-term care insurance was developed by private insurance companies to meet the long-term and chronic health care needs of older adults.

■ Long-term care insurance was designed to pay for long-term health services when multiple chronic health problems occur that require custodial care not covered by Medicare or other insurance.

■ There are many advantages to owning a long-term care insurance policy. However, while insurance companies that offer long-term care policies are usually very ethical, they are essentially businesses with an interest in profit.

- Monthly premiums vary depending on one's age at the time of policy purchase, the length of coverage desired, the waiting period, and the desired amount of daily payments for health care expenses. Premiums are usually not fixed and may increase throughout the coverage period.

- In some cases, the premium may rise so high that older adults are no longer able to afford to pay. This may result in policy cancellation and loss of all previous monthly premiums, just when the policy benefits are needed to cover long-term nursing home, assisted living, or home care services.

- Long-term care insurance generally provides coverage for approved care in nursing facilities and assisted living.

- Care in the home by health care providers and community-based services such as care at adult day care centers are usually covered. Because the policies vary greatly, some services in these facilities may not be covered by long-term care policies.

- Long-term care insurance may be appropriate for middle-income individuals and couples who have too many financial assets to qualify for Medicaid but not enough assets to pay for long-term care.

- Because it has not been available until recently, most of the current cohort of the older adult population would be charged high premiums for coverage. Thus, long-term care insurance is rarely used for paying for long-term health care among today's older adults.

- As baby boomers begin to consider their retirement years and plan for the future, the ability to purchase long-term care insurance and utilize it for payment of future health care expenses will increase.

Veteran's Benefits

- The Department of Veterans Affairs (VA) is a government entity that provides health care for veterans (military personnel who fought during a war).

- VA health care is provided through a network of VA medical centers, hospitals, and health facilities located across the country.

- Once eligibility has been determined, qualified veterans may receive health care for low or no cost.

- Eligibility for VA health care coverage, or the amount of coverage the veteran is entitled to, depends on several factors.

- Most active-duty military personnel who served in the Army, Navy, Air Force, Marines, or Coast Guard and were honorably discharged are eligible for VA health care coverage.

- Military reservists and National Guard members who served on active duty on order from the federal government may also be eligible for some VA health services.

- Eligibility for health care coverage is not limited to those who served in combat.

- The Veterans' Health Care Eligibility Reform Act of 1996 was developed to clarify eligibility for VA health care coverage and improve health benefits for qualified beneficiaries.

- The legislation resulted in the development of the current Uniform Benefits Package—a standard health benefits plan generally available to all veterans.

- Once eligibility has been approved, VA health coverage under the Uniform Benefits Package is comprehensive and provides for both inpatient and outpatient coverage at VA medical centers and facilities nationwide and abroad.

- Outpatient clinics provide physician services, primary and preventive care, diagnostic testing (including laboratory tests), minor surgery, and other needed benefits such as prescription medications.

- The VA will also pay for hearing aids and other services after a small deductible has been met. This service is available even if the prescriptions were written by a physician other than at the VA hospital or facility.

- Veterans with service-connected health problems are usually given priority status; however, because all veterans may receive health care at these clinics, waiting times for appointments and services may be long.

REFERENCES

Alexander, R. (Ed.). (2005). *Avoiding fraud when buying long-term care insurance: A guide for consumers and their families.* Retrieved November 3, 2010, from http://www.alexanderinjury.com/library/library_fraud_1.shtml

Centers for Medicare, & Medicaid Services. (2005). *Medicaid: A brief overview.* Retrieved May 12, 2005, from http://www.cms.hhs.gov/publications/overview-medicare-medicaid/default4.asp

Sale, D. (1996). Standards of care. In D. Sale (Ed.), *Quality assurance* (pp. 37–69). London: MacMillan Press.

Schmadl, J. C. (1979). Quality assurance: Examination of the concept. *Nursing Outlook, 27*(7), 462–465.

Sultz, H. A., & Young, K. M. (1999). *Health care USA* (2nd ed.). Gaithersburg, MD: Aspen.

TEST QUESTIONS

1. One of the most influential advocacy groups for older adults is

   A. The centers for Medicare and Medicaid services

   B. AARP

   C. Association on Aging

   D. Gerontological Society of America

2. Despite improvements in the health care delivery system, older adults do not always receive health care because

   A. They do not want it

   B. They convince themselves that they do not need it

   C. They are afraid of the consequences of illness and treatment

   D. They cannot afford it.

3. Mrs. James is a 71-year-old woman who is entering the hospital for a hip replacement. In counseling her before admission, you know that the primary source of payment for older adult health care is

   A. Medicare

   B. Medicaid

   C. Private insurance

   D. Medigap

4. GNP's role in quality improvement projects may include one of the following:

   A. Identifying standards of care

   B. Articulate a trend in patient care problems

   C. Select the best evidence and implement it into clinical practice

   D. All of the above

5. A health care insurance for older adults that is funded and regulated by the Federal government is entitled

   A. Medicare

   B. Medicaid

   C. Private insurance

   D. Medigap

6. A health care insurance for older adults that is funded and regulated by the State government is entitled

   A. Medicare

   B. Medicaid

   C. Private insurance

   D. Medigap

7. Nurse Practitioners who provide services to Medicare clients receive which of the following percentages of the usual customary and reasonable (UCR) rate of reimbursement?

   A. 20%

   B. 50%

   C. 80%

   D. 100%

8. Hospital insurance for Medicare recipients is funded under

   A. Medicare A

   B. Medicaid A

   C. Medicare B

   D. Medicaid B

9. A health care insurance available for purchase by older adults to help pay for health care needs not paid for by Medicare is

   A. Medicare

   B. Medicaid

   C. Private insurance

   D. Medigap

10. An example of a GNP skill in relation to quality improvement and safety of patients would be

   A. Setting appropriate quality improvement goals

   B. Ensuring patient's rights are protected during quality improvement processes

   C. Assisting in the identification of appropriate quality improvement outcomes

   D. All of the above

11. The greatest source of funding for health care services for America's indigent population is

   A. Medicare

   B. Medicaid

   C. Private insurance

   D. Medigap

12. The Balanced Budget Act of 1997 had one of the following main effects on reimbursement of care for older adults:

   A. Changed Medicare from being a private insurer to managed care.

   B. Restored funds for Medicare

   C. Restored funds for Social Security

   D. Transferred funds from Social Security to Medicare

13. Mrs. Crotwell is a 90-year-old woman who has been hospitalized with a medical diagnosis of osteoporosis. Which of the following is most likely her primary form of insurance?

   A. COBRA

   B. Medicare

   C. Medicaid

   D. HUSKY

14. Which one of the following forms of health care financing is termed *welfare?*

A. Medicare

B. Medicaid

C. Large group insurance

D. COBRA

15. Medicare and Medicaid legislation is an example of which of the following periods in our health care history?

A. 1940s–1950s.

B. 1960s–1970s.

C. 1980s–1990s.

D. 1990s–2000s.

8

Research Utilization

Graduates of GNP programs are all familiar with the nursing research process. However, despite the education that occurs in nursing programs surrounding research, every member of the nursing staff can readily identify examples of outdated clinical practice that is not reflective of currently available nursing research. Unfortunately, many nurses and nurse practitioners do not understand or value research and are more comfortable doing things the way they have "always been done." In fact, many GNPs would be at a loss to provide the scientific rationale behind many common nursing practices, such as application of restraints to keep older adults from falling. The response to why this commonly used practice is being done would likely be "because we have always done it."

The effective utilization of nursing research relies on many factors, including nurses' understanding of the research and evidence-based practice as well as administrative support for research integration. However, regardless of the model used to guide the integration of research into practice, most researchers agree that the first step requires members of the health care team to question current practice. GNPs play an instrumental role in the integration of best evidence into clinical practice across environments of care and are key change agents in promoting quality of care best on best supported research evidence. This chapter will provide an overview of the research process with emphasis on the clinical integration of evidence-based practice. The facilitators and limitations for research utilization and evidence-based practice will be discussed. GNP participation in the research process will also be reviewed. The chapter will conclude with a summary of tips for successful integration of nursing research into clinical practice.

Overview of the Research Process

Nursing research is a process that impacts all members of society. The general target for nursing research initiatives are patients within the health care system. In fact, most nursing research is directed toward improving patient outcomes. However, many others benefit from the nursing research process. GNPs themselves often reap the rewards of research as patient outcomes are improved and the systems used to deliver those outcomes are enhanced. Patient families also may be the direct recipients of nursing research outcomes but also benefit from improved outcomes of patients. Other members of the interdisciplinary team also benefit from the outcomes of nursing research. Finally, nursing research provides the opportunity to enhance the cost-effectiveness of care, which in turn saves the government and taxpayer's money.

Research means to "search again" and is defined as a diligent and systematic inquiry into a targeted area or problem. It results in the discovery of new knowledge to improve patient outcomes. Nursing research is conducted in a variety of clinical settings in which patients are cared. These include home care, nursing homes, hospitals, clinics, and assisted living communities. Nursing research may also be conducted in a laboratory setting and then applied later directly to practice.

Research in nursing is critically important as it is the foundation of new knowledge in nursing. The information we now have to care for patients was not available 50 years ago. In fact, all we know about nursing was generated through the research nurses and other members of the health care profession. The priorities for nursing research are to improve the following:

■ Nursing as a profession

■ Nursing practice

■ Patient outcomes

Before starting any new research project and critical to all evidence-based practice projects, the GNP must conduct a literature review. The purpose of the literature review is to explore the following:

■ What is known and not known about a subject

■ Gaps, consistencies, and inconsistencies in the literature about a subject

■ Unanswered questions about the subject

There are two main methods of nursing research: qualitative and quantitative. Qualitative research is often considered subjective and quantitative is considered objective. Qualitative research focuses on the collection of data through interviews, observations and focuses groups to enhance understanding about a particular area of interest in nursing. Examples of qualitative research designs include phenomenological research, grounded theory research, ethnographic research, and historical research. General approaches to data collection for qualitative studies include focus groups, interviews, and observation. Approaches to qualitative research are as follows:

■ Phenomenology: both a philosophy and a research method. The purpose is to describe experiences as they are lived and to capture the "lived experience" of study participants.

■ Grounded theory is based on symbolic interaction theory and holds many views in common with phenomenology. It explores how people define reality and how their beliefs are related to their actions.

■ Ethnographic research is developed by anthropologists as a mechanism for studying cultures. The word *ethnographic* means "portrait of a people." This research method seeks to understand people—ways of living, believing, and adapting.

■ Historical research examines events of the past to enhance self-understanding.

Quantitative research gathers data in numerical form through responses to objective questionnaires (such as the State-Trait Anxiety Inventory, Spielberg, 1983) or collection of physiological measures such as blood pressure, pulse, or laboratory values. Approaches to data collection for quantitative studies include collection of objective biophysiological data and surveys. There are a number of different types of quantitative research designs such as descriptive research, quasi-experimental research, and experimental research. These research designs are defined below:

■ Descriptive Research: Research aimed to systematically describe a particular situation or event. The findings are generally provided using descriptive statistics such as mean, median, mode, standard deviation, and range.

■ Correlational Research: Explores the relationship between two or more variables.

■ Experimental Research: Research aimed at determining the effect of one or more variable(s) (independent variable) on one or more dependent variables. An example of this may be a research study that measures the impact of a nursing intervention, such as a fall prevention program on the number of falls among older adults. For a true experimental design to exist, the following conditions must be met: (1) the sample must be randomly selected, (2) there must be manipulation of the independent variable by the researcher as is usually seen in intervention studies and (3) there must be a control group.

■ Quasi experimental Research: This research method is similar to the experimental method but lacks usually a random sample and/or control condition.

- Longitudinal Research: This research method may follow any of the designs that are mentioned previously but follows the same research subjects over a period of time, generally greater than 1 year.

- Cross-sectional Research: May also assume a number of research designs but only collects data at one point in time, with no follow-up.

In quantitative research in which research instruments are used, it is essential to ensure that the instruments possess reliability (see Table 8.1) and validity (see Table 8.2). Reliability refers to the instrument's ability to consistently measure a variable. Validity refers to an instrument's ability to measure what it is supposed to measure.

The criteria for determining reliability and validity of research instruments are listed in Tables 8.1 and 8.2.

Nursing research is always guided by theory. Theory is a systematic, abstract explanation of some aspect of reality. In most cases, nursing theory is used to guide nursing research. There are two types of nursing theories to guide research: nursing grand theories and middle-range nursing theories. Nursing theory is a group of related concepts that guide practice. It is abstract (not measurable) and an essential component of professional knowledge base (all professionals must have theoretical base). It is made of four concepts:

- Person

- Environment

- Nursing

- Health

Nursing grand theories are abstract, connect and relate the four main concepts, are not generally measurable, and are not always easily adapted to nursing research. Following are examples of nursing grand theories:

- Nightingale (1859) enhancing body's reparative processes by manipulation of noise, nutrition, hygiene, light, comfort, socialization, and hope

TABLE 8.1

Criteria for Determining Reliability of a Research Instrument

Type	Measure	Statistic
Test-retest	Participants completed questionnaire similarly on two separate attempts.	Correlation (r)
Inter-rater	Two or more people who administered an instrument came up with similar scores.	Correlation (r)
Internal Consistency	Items of an instrument correlate well with other items on the instrument.	Alpha Coefficient (a)

TABLE 8.2

Criteria for Determining Validity of a Research Instrument

Type	Definition	Statistic	Note
Content Validity	Developed by individuals with established expertise in the content	None	Conducted while instrument is being developed
Construct Validity	Items in the instrument group with similar concepts which were consistent with the purpose of the tool.	Item Analysis	Conducted while instrument is being developed
Face Validity	Evaluated by experts as appearing to be appropriate	None	Conducted before or after the instrument has been developed; is of little value
Criterion Validity	Results of this tool were correctly predicted by the results of another tool.	Regression	Conducted after the instrument has been developed to determine its usefulness for a particular study
Convergent Validity	Results of this tool correlate positively with similar items on a similar tool.	Positive Correlation	Conducted after the instrument has been developed to determine its usefulness for a particular study
Discriminant Validity	Results of this tool correlate negatively with opposite items on an opposite tool.	Negative Correlation	Conducted after the instrument has been developed to determine its usefulness for a particular study; may only be used when clearly opposite concepts are found in an instrument

- Benner and Wrubel (1989) caring as a means of coping with the stressors of illness; caring is central to the essence of nursing

- Orem (1971) caring and helping clients to attain total self care

- King (1971) communication to help clients reestablish positive adaptation to the environment. Supports that the nursing process is defined as dynamic interpersonal process between nurse, client and health systems

- Watson (1979) promoting health, restoring the client to health, and preventing illness

- Roy and Andrews (1999) identifying types of demands placed on the client, assessing adaptation to demands, and helping clients adapt. Adaptation model is based on physiological, psychological, and sociological adaptive roles.

- Neuman (1982) assisting individuals, families, and groups in attaining and maintaining maximal level of total wellness by purposeful interventions. Stress reduction is the goal of the theory.

- Leininger (1991) transcultural theory works as a unifying domain for nursing knowledge and practice, providing care consistent with nursing's emerging science and knowledge with caring as a central focus.

- Henderson (1966) focuses on the need to work independently with other health care workers assisting the client to gain independence as quickly as possible.

- Peplau (1952) developing interaction between nurse and client

- Rogers (1970) maintaining and promoting health, preventing illness, and care for and rehabilitate ill and disabled clients through humanistic science of nursing to help people develop into unitary human beings

- Abdellah, Beland, Martin, and Matheney (1960) providing service to individuals, families, and society to be kind and caring but also intelligent, competent, and technically well prepared to provide this service and involves 21 nursing problems

Nursing middle-range theories are used far more often to provide a framework for nursing research then nursing grand theories. Middle-range theories are defined as those "that lie between the minor but necessary working hypotheses that evolve in abundance during day-to-day research and all-inclusive, systematic efforts to develop unified theory" (Merton, 1968, p. 9). There are many middle-range theories both from nursing and related disciplines that guide nursing research. Liehr and Smith (1999) provide eight main categories of middle-range theory as described below.

- Community empowerment is related to participatory action research with the underlying belief that to improve the health of a community, members of the community must take responsibility for and actively participate in health-related interventions and programming.

- Family stress and adaptation theories stem from sociological theory and have evolved extensively over the past century. It includes coping, stress, and resiliency models. The theory supports that effective family response to stress in the form of the development of new or existing resources for coping and stress management.

- Meaning middle-range theory has roots in the psychological discipline. There are three major components of the theory: life purpose, freedom to choose, and human suffering. A number of psychological instruments and interventions have been developed by nursing and related disciplines to facilitate the process of purpose and meaning throughout the lifespan.

- Self-efficacy is the confidence or belief in one's capabilities to organize and execute the courses of action required to produce given outcomes (Bandura, 1997). Self efficacy is an important concept in self-management and reflects one's ability to perform a behavior or task. Self-efficacy refers to the patient's confidence that he or she can manage symptoms and distress. Self-efficacy is an important variable in understanding adjustment to disease, and psychoeducational interventions that provide information and support may increase self-efficacy in both patients and their caregivers.

- Self-transcendence relies on the full realization of human potential throughout life. It focuses on the ability to attain well-being, while being vulnerable to personal mortality. The theory is heavily used during care of older adults and patients till the end of life.

- Story theory focuses on the ability of the patient to tell their life story and that of others involved in their life and health care in efforts to successfully adapt, cope, and transcend. It is a process rather than outcome theory, which is used widely for patients coping with numerous health and illness situations.

- Uncertainty theory was proposed by Mishel (1988) and supports the idea that the nature of chronic illness causes continual uncertainty to spread from uncertainty about symptoms and disease state to uncertainty about broader life issues and the ability to achieve valued goals. Meaning attached to usual routines is disrupted. The disruption or intrusiveness of the event caused by continued uncertainty can dismantle a person's sense of order and structure. Research surrounding this theory has focused on interventions to reduce uncertainty in patients across the illness spectrum.

- Unpleasant symptoms theory is applicable to many patient situations in which patients experience unpleasant symptoms in response to illness or treatment. This is a newer theory developed over the past decade that is increasing in popularity for its ability to provide a framework to manage outcomes of pain, dyspnea, nausea, vomiting, and fatigue.

GNP Role in Research and Evidence-Based Practice

The first step to successful implementation of best research into clinical practice is identifying a clinical problem or realizing that there may be new information available which leads GNPs to question current clinical practice. In general, for GNPs to effectively utilize nursing research, they have to identify that new information is available and value the role of that information in changing practice. Sometimes the best research never makes it into clinical practice. Following are some of the ways in which researchers can facilitate the integration of their research into practice:

1. Minimize research and statistical jargon as much as possible.

2. Emphasize the clinical application of the research.

3. Present the findings at a research and evidence-based practice conferences.

4. Publish the article in a highly-read nursing journal.

Closs and Cheater (1994) suggest that both interest and education are essential to change attitudes toward the role of research in clinical practice. Nurses may not always read research reports and value the role of nursing research in clinical practice. In many cases, nurses have not experienced the positive impact of research on patient care. Practice change may be stimulated by reading information that may be immediately applicable to improving practice. To generate an interest and appreciation for research among GNPs and staff nurses, it is essential that nurses are aware that new pieces of evidence are currently being used clinically. Involvement of the entire patient care staff is essential to facilitate evidence-based practice change. Attendance at professional nursing conferences, in which research information is shared, is an excellent way of generating interest, improving attitudes, and raising levels of excitement among GNPs.

The availability of Internet-based search engines facilitates the searching of evidence, once a practice problem has been identified. Evidence-based practice relies on direct sources of nursing research. The most popular sources for this literature are the Cumulative Index to Nursing and Allied Health Literature (CINAHL) and MEDLINE.

Access to the information contained in these databases requires both membership and payment on an individual or institutional level. It is essential that GNPs have access to these Internet-based databases to obtain information to guide evidence-based practice.

Evaluation and synthesis of available research evidence is the next essential step toward evidence-based practice. One research article on a topic rarely provides the evidence for practice change. It is necessary for GNPs to critically review all relevant literature on the topic at hand and present a synthesis of the findings to begin integrating the best evidence into practice. This may occur in a number of ways. The GNP can review all the articles and develop a grid with a summary of findings and a ranking of the evidence that can be reviewed by the practice change team.

For research to be valuable for patient care, the research must be used. Efforts toward evidence-based practice or "the integration of clinical expertise with the best available external clinical Internet-acquired evidence from systematic research" (Sackett, Rosenberg, Gray, Haynes, & Richardson, 1996) is prevalent in nursing and other clinical arenas. However, integration of the best research evidence into practice requires access to the best research evidence and the ability to determine what the best evidence is and which is not. Nurse Practitioners must become educated consumers of nursing research to understand the evidence which should be integrated into nursing practice. Table 8.3 provides some common grading systems used by the U.S. Preventative Services Task Force that may be helpful in determining what evidence should be integrated into clinical practice.

Finally, successful integration of nursing research into practice requires removal of institutional barriers. Organizational characteristics identified as barriers to research utilization include available facilities and cooperation of the nursing and interdisciplinary staff. It is only when GNPs acknowledge that practice needs to change, access appropriate knowledge to make that change, and can successfully change practice, the evidence-based practice occurs. It is essential that nursing administration develop a research capacity within clinical environments. Such an environment allows the free questioning of existing nursing practice and openness to new approaches to health care. Within such environments, GNPs can lead journal clubs and research committees, facilitate research and evidence-based practice presentations, as well as support opportunities to participate in these activities outside the workplace. GNPs can be the advocates for advanced software search systems, online nursing journals, and small grants to facilitate evidence-based practice projects. GNPs can also function as the leader in facilitating interdisciplinary partnerships between and among clinicians, researchers, and administrators to facilitate the identification of clinical problems, information seeking, and integration into the clinical area.

The GNP can also assist in creating an environment of change. Regardless of how effectively the problem has been articulated and the literature searched and synthesized, change presents risk and is associated with fear of the unknown. However, regardless of the risk, change must be allowed

TABLE 8.3

U.S. Preventative Services Task Force Grading Criteria for Evidence-Based Practice

1. Strength of Recommendation

   1. Rating A: Good Evidence to Support

   2. Rating B: Fair Evidence to Support

   3. Rating D: Fair Evidence Against

   4. Rating E: Good Evidence Against

2. Quality of Evidence

   1. Level I

      1. Evidence from 1 or more randomized controlled trials

   2. Level II-1

      1. Evidence from controlled trials, but no randomization

3. Level II-2

   1. Evidence from cohort or case-control studies

4. Level II-3

   1. Evidence from multiple time or historic controls

5. Level III

   1. Expert opinion based on clinical experience

Reference: (1996). USPSTF Clinical Preventative Services (2nd ed.). *http://www.fpnotebook.com/Prevent/Epi/UsPrvntvSrvcsTskFrcRcmndtns.htm*

to happen for evidence to be effectively integrated into clinical practice. The successful integration of currently available research into clinical areas is essential to create an environment of evidence-based practice. However, the literature shows that many barriers remain to the creating of evidence-based practice settings. The following tips, adapted from Cheater and Closs (1994), may be helpful in promoting evidence-based practice in clinical settings.

■ Develop a "climate of opinion" in which research is valued and appreciated as an integral part of clinical practice, by challenging practice in nonthreatening manner.

■ Demonstrate how evidence is currently being used clinically.

■ Lead a team to select a prevalent practice problem and together review the literature, decide on a practice plan, and implement it. If something saves the health care team time and improves patient outcomes, it is likely to be implemented.

- Ensure that members of the health care team have access to research evidence and know how to use available databases.

- Promote administrative support for the use of evidence-based practice with certificates, promotions, and acknowledgement.

ETHICAL ISSUES IN RESEARCH

Research on human subjects requires adherence to ethical principles and protection of human rights. Ethical principles include the following:

- Principle of beneficence (do no harm)
  - Freedom from harm
  - Freedom from exploitation
- Principle of respect for human dignity
  - Right to self-determination
  - Right to full disclosure
- Principle of justice
  - Right to fair treatment
  - Right to privacy

Review and approval of research proposals by respective Institutional Review Boards (IRBs) before the initiation of any research project is the most effective manner to protect the rights of human subjects. To ensure that patient's rights to the self-determination are protected, most research studies require that patients sign informed consent documents before the involvement in research projects. Even older adults who have cognitive impairment must give informed consent to participate in research. If older adults have a conservator, this person may give informed consent in the place of the research participant. However, the patient should still be fully informed of the research study and should not be forced to participate if they are reluctant in any way.

Summary and Conclusion

The GNPs involvement in research primarily involves the integration of best evidence into clinical practice. However, to do this, the GNP must first be aware of what is good research, the barriers to research utilization, and methods to overcome these barriers. The GNP will utilize research knowledge to participate in unit and institutional research projects and quality improvement efforts. With knowledge of good research practices, the GNP is ideally qualified to facilitate evidence-based practice, while protecting the rights of human subjects.

REFERENCES

Abdellah, F. G., Beland, I. L., Martin, A., & Matheney, R. V. (1960). *Patient-centered approaches to nursing*. New York: Macmillan.

Bandura, A. (1997). *Self-efficacy: The exercise of control*. New York: W.H. Freeman.

Benner, P., & Wrubel, J. (1989). *The primacy of caring: Stress and coping in health and illness*. Kent, OH: Addison-Wesley.

Closs, S. J., & Cheater, F. M. (1994). Utilization of nursing research: Culture, interest and support. *Journal of Advanced Nursing, 19*, 762–773.

Henderson, V. (1966). *The nature of nursing*. New York: Macmillan.

King, I. M. (1971). *Toward a theory for nursing: General concepts of human behavior*. New York: John Wiley & Sons.

Leininger, M. (1991). Transcultural nursing: The study and practice field. *Imprint, 38*(2), 55–66.

Liehr, P., & Smith, M. J. (1999). Middle range theory: Spinning research and practice to create knowledge for the new millennium. *Advances in Nursing Science, 21*(4), 81–91.

Merton, R. K. (1968). On sociological theories of the middle range. In R. K. Merton (Ed.), *Social theory and social structure* (pp. 39–72). New York: Free Press.

Neuman, B. (1982). The systems concept and nursing. In B. Neuman (Ed.), *The Neuman systems model: Application to nursing education and practice* (pp. 3–7). Norwalk, CT: Appleton-Century-Crofts.

Mishel, M. H. (1988). Uncertainty in illness. *Image: Journal of Nursing Scholarship, 20*, 225–232.

Nightingale, F. (1859). *Notes on nursing: what it is and what it is not* [With an introduction by Barbara Stevens Barnum and commentaries by contemporary nursing leaders. 1992, Commemorative edition]. Philadelphia: J.B. Lippingcott Company.

Orem, D. E. (1971) *Nursing: Concepts of practice*. New York: McGraw-Hill

Peplau, H. E. (1952). *Interpersonal relations in nursing*. New York: G.P. Putnam's Sons.

Rogers, M. E. (1970). *An introduction to the theoretical basis of nursing*. Philadelphia: FA Davis.

Roy, C., & Andrews, H. (1999). *The Roy adaptation model* (2nd ed.). Stamford, CT: Appleton & Lange.

Sackett, D. L., Rosenberg, W. M., Gray, J. A., Haynes, R. B., & Richardson, WS. (1996). Evidence-based medicine: What it is and what it isn't. *British Medical Journal, 312*, 71–72.

Spielberg, C. D., *Manual for the State-Trait Anxiety Inventory (STAI)*. 1983, Palo Alto, CA: Consulting Psychologists Press.

Watson, J. (l979). *Nursing: The philosophy and science of caring*. Boston: Little, Brown and Company. 2nd printing 1985, Boulder, CO: University Press of Colorado. Translated into French, Korean.

TEST QUESTIONS

1. A GNP observes that older adult patients of a nursing home show behavior changes in the early evening. She would like to know more about this phenomenon. The GNP wants to believe it is important to work with a research method that explores and describes everyday experiences to generate and enhance the understanding of what it means to be human. What would be the most appropriate research method?

    A. Grounded theory

    B. Longitudinal

    C. Ethnographic

    D. Phenomenological

2. To develop an evidence-based practice project on a research unit, the GNP must first conduct a literature review. All of the following are purposes of the literature review for this study, except:

    A. Determining what is known and not known about a subject

    B. Determining gaps, consistencies, and inconsistencies in the literature about a subject

    C. Discovering unanswered questions about the subject

    D. Determining the most appropriate method of disseminating the research

3. A GNP is working on a research study that is testing a medication (Celluex) on the long-term impact on blood pressure of all patients on a cardiac unit at her hospital. How would you describe the study design used in this case?

    A. Descriptive, cross sectional

    B. Experimental, longitudinal

    C. Quasi experimental, longitudinal

    D. Experimental, cross sectional

4. If the researcher is interested in selecting a middle-range theory to support this research, which theory would be the most appropriate?

   A. Roy Adaptation theory

   B. Self-efficacy theory

   C. Neuman's stress reduction theory

   D. Transcultural nursing theory

5. If the GNP was interested in developing an instrument to measure the subtle symptoms of hypertension exhibited by subjects in this study and wanted to test it to make sure it measured what it was supposed to measure, what would she be testing for?

   A. Reliability

   B. Velocity

   C. Heterogeneity

   D. Validity

6. A GNP is concerned that patient care assistants are not as prepared to provide assistance with Activities of Daily Living (ADLs) than RNs, in geriatric care units. She decides to send out a preparedness questionnaire to PCAs and RNs who work in geriatric care units of a particular hospital. How would you describe the data collection method used in this study?

   A. Quantitative/survey method

   B. Quantitative/biophysiological methods

   C. Qualitative/interview method

   D. Qualitative/participant observation

7. The GNP finds that RNs are more prepared than PCAs to provide assistance with ADLs. All the following methods will help her to present her findings with as few barriers to research utilization as possible, *except*:

   A. Minimize research and statistical jargon as much as possible.

   B. Emphasize the clinical application of the research.

   C. Present the findings at a conference usually attended by only nurse researchers.

   D. Publish the article in a highly-read nursing journal.

8. Sometimes research is not utilized, despite its quality. All the following reasons may explain the prevention of research utilization, *except* when:

   A. Nurses were not taught to understand research in nursing school.

   B. Nurses don't always read research reports.

   C. Nurses, as a group, feel research is useless.

   D. The positive impact of research on patient care is not observed when applied.

9. A nurse researcher is interested in discovering the reasons why centenarians (people who live to be 100 years old or older) live so long. She decides to use open-ended interviews over a 5 year period on nine centenarians, hand-picked to participate in the study. What research method was used in this study?

   A. Experimental

   B. Quasi experimental

   C. Longitudinal

   D. Correlational

10. What problem would the researcher *most* likely encounter because of the sampling and design?

    A. Unsupported reliability of the research instrument

    B. Lack of literature on the topic of interest

    C. Difficulty gaining human subjects' approval

    D. Attrition of the sample

11. How would the researcher protect the patient's right to self-determination in a research study?

    A. Obtaining only quantitative/objective data

    B. Obtaining informed consent

    C. Obtaining qualitative/interviews

    D. Using qualitative/participant observation techniques

12. The chosen research method seeks to explore and describe the experience of centenarians. This method is best described as:

    A. Grounded theory

    B. Longitudinal

    C. Ethnographic

    D. Phenomenological

13. Which of the following ethical principles that the researcher must uphold means do no harm?

    A. Principle of beneficence

    B. Principle of respect for human dignity

    C. Principle of justice

    D. Principle of privacy

14. In selecting a middle-range theory to support a research project, which of the following should the GNP include?

    A. Roger's Science of Unitary Human Beings

    B. Mishel's Uncertainty in Illness model

    C. Orem's Theory of Caring

    D. Roy's Adaptation model

15. In preparing the Institutional Review Board Application, it is essential to include one of the following elements to ensure patient's rights to self-determination:

    A. Informed consent

    B. Conclusions

    C. Purpose

    D. Participant's names

Gerontological Nurse Practitioner Comprehensive Test

1. A 72-year-old man at the adult day care center states that he cannot have a flu shot because last time it made him get the flu. The best response by the NP would be

   A. "The influenza vaccine is capable of giving you osteoarthritis, but not the flu."

   B. "The influenza vaccine is made of a live attenuated virus and is not capable of giving you the flu."

   C. "The influenza vaccine is made of inactivated (dead) virus and is not capable of giving you the flu."

   D. "This is possible, but the risks of getting sick and dying from the flu are greater than your risk of getting the virus from the vaccine."

2. Mr. Smith, a 92-year-old man, has had the flu several times and has received annual flu vaccinations for the past 10 years. This year, there is a shortage of influenza vaccinations, and he states he is probably already immune and should let his wife have his vaccine as she needs it more. Your best response would be

   A. "The process of antigenic shift causes small changes in the virus that happens continually over time, producing new virus strains that may not be recognized by his body's immune system."

   B. "The process of antigenic drift causes abrupt, major changes in the virus resulting in new viruses that may not be recognized by his body's immune system."

   C. Both A and B

   D. "As an older adult, you are still in the high-priority group for vaccination."

3. Ms. Singer, a 76-year-old healthy female residing alone at home, presents to your clinic this winter season with classic flu symptoms (high fever, cough, nausea, and fatigue) about the 3rd day since feeling poorly. Essential data necessary to develop a diagnosis and plan of care include

   A. Nasal secretions for culture and sensitivity

   B. History and physical exam findings

   C. Chest x-ray

   D. Pulmonary function test results

4. The best treatment choice for Ms. Singer in the previous question would be

   A. Symmetrel (Amantadine) 100 mg Bid × 5 days

   B. Flumadine (Rimantadine) 100 mg BID × 5 days

   C. Zanamavir (Relenza) 450 mg × 10 days

   D. Rest and increased fluid intake

5. Mr. B was exposed to TB 1 week ago by a visiting relative diagnosed with active TB. The patient's last PPD was negative. He is not in a high-risk group. The result of the PPD planted 72 hours ago is 10-mm induration. You tell Mr. B that

   A. "The test is negative now; you need to be tested again in 3 months to confirm that this exposure did not infect you."

   B. "The test is positive for TB; you should begin immediate treatment for TB exposure."

   C. "The test showed no TB infection; you should continue with annual monitoring by PPD."

   D. "The test is positive for TB; you should have a chest x-ray immediately to determine the extent of infection."

6. The definitive test for diagnosing active TB is

   A. Forced vital capacity (FCV)

   B. Sputum culture for acid fast bacillus

   C. PPD (Mantoux test)

   D. Chest x-ray

7. Mr. Miller is a 65-year-old patient who presents with a 2-week history of malaise, headache, nasal congestion, myalgia, and sore throat. He has felt more and more exhausted over the past week and has missed 2 days of work. He thinks he has had a high fever, and last night had chills, and waking this morning in a sweat. His cough is moderately productive of "greenish" sputum. His appetite has been poor, but he is drinking fluids and does not feel he has lost any weight since he has been sick. He admits to a 2-ppd cigarette habit, starting at the age of 15. Given this information, the most likely differential diagnosis is

   A. Bronchitis

   B. URI

   C. Pneumonia

   D. COPD

8. Other important historical information that may help to make a diagnosis in Mr. Miller's case from the previous question includes

   A. Past history of STDs

   B. Occupation as a teacher

   C. History of concomitant immunocompromised

   D. History of headaches

9. When conducting the physical exam on Mr. Miller from the previous question, the NP would expect to find

   A. Decreased respiratory rate and dullness to percussion

   B. Dullness to percussion and adventitious sounds

   C. Decreased respiratory rate and adventitious lung sounds

   D. Increased respiratory rate and pleural friction rub.

10. Which of the following tests measures the amount of actively replicating HIV virus and correlates with the disease progression and response to antiviral drugs?

   A. Western blot

   B. HIV viral load test

   C. Absolute CD4 lymphocyte count

   D. CD4 Lymphocyte percentage

11. Mr. Moran, a 69-year-old man, presents to the clinic with possible HIV infection. The three most common signs and symptoms of early, primary HIV infection are

    A. Weight loss, pharyngitis, and fatigue

    B. Fever, fatigue, and pharyngitis

    C. Joint pain, confusion, and fever

    D. Numbness, nausea, and fever

12. Mrs. Falcone, a 72-year-old patient, has been diagnosed with multi-drug resistant TB (MDR TB). Appropriate treatments for her would most likely include

    A. Isoniazid (INH)

    B. Rifampin (Rifadin)

    C. Pyrazinamide

    D. Gentamicin

13. The patient is said to have AIDS when he or she has a:

    A. CD4 count less than 200, no symptoms of HIV

    B. CD4 count more than 200, opportunistic infections

    C. CD4 count less than 200, opportunistic infections

    D. CD4 count less than 200, viral load less than 10,000

14. Mr. Packard has been diagnosed with community-acquired pneumonia (CAP). As the NP working in the primary care clinic, you know that the most common pathogen that causes this type of pneumonia is

    A. *Streptococcus pneumoniae*

    B. *Legionella*

    C. *M. tuberculosis*

    D. *H. influenza*

15. You are an NP in an HIV clinic; a client with HIV infection has a CD4 count of 200 and an HIV viral load of 75. The client is asymptomatic. The patient is currently homeless. As the NP, what is your next course of action?

    A. Discuss treating with HIV antiretrovirals when patient becomes symptomatic and plan is made for storing and administration of medication.

    B. Defer treatment until CD4 count goes below 50 and plan is made for storing and administration of medication.

    C. Initiate treatment as soon as a plan is made for the storing and administration of medication.

    D. Repeat CD4 and viral load tests before initiating treatment.

16. Mrs. Stacy is about to begin her series of hepatitis B vaccinations. The NP tests her for a serological marker, and the results show the hepatitis B surface antibody (HbsAb). This tells you that Mrs. Stacy

    A. Needs to begin the series as soon as possible

    B. Needs to have a repeat blood test because this one reading is not indicative of immunity

    C. Has an active hepatitis B infection

    D. Is immune to hepatitis B

17. Chronic hepatitis B is diagnosed when

    A. Liver cancer develops

    B. Liver biopsy has hepatitis B virus

    C. Hepatitis B surface antigen is positive $\geq$ 6 months

    D. Hepatitis B immune globulin M is present

18. The causative agent of hepatitis A is excreted from the body primarily through

    A. Skin

    B. Feces

    C. Urine

    D. Blood

19. Your 81-year-old patient reveals that she is interested in becoming sexually active with a man who has recently been diagnosed with hepatitis B. She has not been vaccinated against hepatitis B and has no prior history of hepatitis B infection. You counsel her to

    A. Receive immune globulin and start hepatitis vaccinations

    B. Start hepatitis B vaccinations

    C. Limit the number of sexual partners

    D. Be tested for HbsAb

20. A 66-year-old man returning from an extended trip to Eastern Europe reported experiencing several-weeks of nausea, vomiting, and lethargy which is gradually resolving. You suspect infection with hepatitis B, but lab values for hepatitis B surface antigen and hepatitis B surface antibodies are negative. Which of the following lab tests would be most helpful in establishing the diagnosis of hepatitis B?

    A. Elevated alkaline phosphatase

    B. IgM antibody to hepatitis B core antigen

    C. Elevated serum AST

    D. Total antibody to hepatitis A

21. The gold standard for the diagnosis of hepatitis C is

    A. HCV RNA

    B. Hepatitis C antibody on ELISA

    C. Anti-HCV enzyme immunoassay

    D. Elevated serum AST

22. The choice of antibiotic for community-acquired pneumonia is

    A. Doxycycline

    B. Gentamicin

    C. Erythromycin

    D. Azithromycin (Zithromax)

23. Mrs. Robert's is a 65-year-old African-American widowed woman who is 5 years postmenopausal. Last week, she began her period and has continued moderate bleeding since this time. She denies recent sexual contact. The most likely cause of this bleeding is

    A. Fibroid tumors

    B. Hypothyroidism

    C. Chronic lymphocytic leukemia

    D. Stein-Leventhal syndrome

24. To diagnose Mrs. Robert's in the previous question, which of the following tests would be most appropriate?

    A. T4 and TSH

    B. MRI

    C. Ultrasound

    D. FSH and LH

25. If Mrs. Robert's is suspected of having endometrial/uterine cancer, which of the following procedures will result in the ability to test the entire uterine lining?

    A. Uterine core biopsy

    B. Uterine ultrasound

    C. Dilation and Curettage (D&C)

    D. Myomectomy

26. When the patient has emphysema, the NP might expect to hear _____ on auscultation.

    A. Wheezes

    B. Increased A/P diameter

    C. Hyperresonance

    D. Coarse crackles

27. The best medication(s) to prescribe for a COPD patient with mild inter-mittent asthma symptoms is

    A. Anticholinergic MDI and oral steroids

    B. Beta-agonist MDI and amoxicillin

    C. Steroids MDI only

    D. Proventil HFA MDI only

28. All of the following are signs of asthma *except*

    A. Edema of bronchial mucosa

    B. Mucus plugging of the airways

    C. Barrel chest

    D. Bronchospasm

29. Chronic obstructive pulmonary disease is characterized by

    A. Cilia production

    B. Significant reduction in expiratory airflow

    C. Erosion of cartilage in the bronchioles

    D. Reversible bronchospasm

30. A 74-year-old female athlete is diagnosed with asthma. Her social activities over the past 3 to 4 weeks seem to have aggravated her condition, but she is able to participate successfully with additional medications. Daily control medication and rescue proventil MDI before sports activity are included in the current management. According to this level of therapy, this case of asthma is classified as

    A. Mild intermittent

    B. Severe persistent

    C. Moderate persistent

    D. Mild persistent

31. Ms. Samuels, a 64-year-old female, recently took a position as a phlebotomist in a community health clinic, and her employer requires her to be immunized against hepatitis B. Your response to this requirement would be to

    A. Check hepatitis B surface antigen for prior immunity and if not immune, vaccinate her against hepatitis B

    B. Vaccinate her against hepatitis B

    C. Give her a letter waiving her from the hepatitis B requirement due to her age.

    D. Give her 1/2 the usual hepatitis B vaccination dose over six immunization periods.

32. Ms. Johnson presents to the primary care practice because she believes she is approaching menopause. To determine if a woman is approaching menopause, the most effective laboratory test would be

    A. Serial LH levels

    B. Single LH level

    C. Serial FSH levels

    D. One-time FSH level

33. Mrs. Johnson is complaining of frequent hot flashes. Hot flashes associated with menopause are generally associated with surges in which hormone?

    A. LH

    B. FSH

    C. Estrogen

    D. Progesterone

34. In attempting to provide teaching to Mrs. Johnson regarding herbal supplements to help with hot flashes, it is important to remember that the only herbal supplement associated with supported effectiveness at reducing hot flashes is

    A. St. John's wort

    B. Black cohosh

    C. Ginseng

    D. Gingko biloba

35. In providing teaching to Ms. Carmen, a 73-year-old menopausal woman, it is important to inform her that the risk factors for osteoporosis include

    A. Diets rich in calcium

    B. BMI more than 22

    C. BMI less than 22

    D. Active lifestyle

36. Mrs. Cecil is an 86-year-old white female who presents with pain related to vertebral fracture secondary to postmenopausal osteoporosis. The most effective medication to treat both her pain and her osteoporosis is

    A. Actonel (risedronate)

    B. Fosamx (aledronate)

    C. Miacalcin (calcitonin)

    D. Boniva (ibandronate)

37. A 73-year-old woman comes to your office complaining of problems swallowing. She says food appears to hang up in her sternal area. This started several years ago and has steadily progressed. Within the last month, she has had symptoms at least twice per week. Generally, only solid foods cause problems. She does not regurgitate food and has a stable weight. What is the symptom this patient is complaining of?

    A. Dysphagia

    B. Angina

    C. GERD

    D. Aerophagia

38. All of the following are true about Barrett's Esophagitis *except*

    A. Males are more likely to have Barrett's than females

    B. Barrett's is because of a change in the esophageal mucosa from columnar to squamous

    C. Barrett's esophagitis occurs in patients with PUD

    D. Patients with Barrett's Esophagitis are under greater risk for a GIB than any other patients who have GERD

39. Walter Bacon is a 98-year-old male complaining of a 3-week history of burning in the epigastric area of the chest. He has had "heartburn" in the past for which he took Tums with relief. This burning is much worse now, and he does not get relief from antacids. Sometimes, he can taste "stomach acid" in his throat. You note that he is overweight. This limited history suggests which of the following differential diagnoses?

  A. Chest pain of cardiac origin

  B. PUD/GERD

  C. COPD

  D. Muscle strain of chest

40. Hyperemia, edema, and erosion of the esophageal luminal surface may result from

  A. Crohn's disease

  B. Appendicitis

  C. Gastroesophageal reflux disease (GERD)

  D. Pernicious anemia

41. Certain foods such as coffee, garlic, and fried foods cause the symptom of GERD because

  A. They weaken the LES tone

  B. They cause constipation

  C. They cause diarrhea

  D. They promote transmission of *H. Pylori*

42. Most cases of peptic ulcer are caused by

  A. Genetic predisposition

  B. Stress

  C. Poor diet

  D. *H. Pylori*

43. Risk factors for *H. Pylori* include all the following *except*

    A. Low socioeconomic status

    B. Obesity

    C. Poor sanitary conditions

    D. Crowded living conditions

44. Treatment for a patient infected with *H. Pylori* consists of

    A. Antacids and antibiotics

    B. PPIs and H2RAs

    C. PPIs and antibiotics

    D. H2RAs and antacids

45. Mr. Diamond is a 69-year-old white male who presents to the primary care practice with normal visual acuity and pupillary responses, and complaints of red, dry, itchy eyes. The most likely cause of his symptoms is

    A. Allergic conjunctivitis

    B. Bacterial conjunctivitis

    C. Iritis

    D. Angle closure glaucoma

46. Mr. Ted is a 69-year-old white male who presents to the primary care practice with new onset reduced visual acuity and fixed dilated pupils. Your course of action would be

    A. Steroid eye drops

    B. Oral steroids

    C. Both oral steroids and steroid eye drops

    D. Immediate referral to opthamologist or Emergency Department

47. Ms. Green is an 82-year-old white female who presents to the primary care practice with normal visual acuity and pupillary responses, no discomfort, and purulent discharge from both eyes. The most likely cause of her symptoms is

    A. Allergic conjunctivitis

    B. Bacterial conjunctivitis

    C. Iritis

    D. Closed angle glaucoma

48. Mr. Paulson is a 78-year-old obese, white male with type II diabetes. His weight is 129 kg. He presents to the primary care practice with 2+ proteinuria and a serum creatinine of 1.8. Which category of renal failure is this patient in?

    A. Stage 1

    B. Stage 2

    C. Stage 3

    D. Stage 4

49. Mr. Paulson's would be considered at greatest risk for nephrotic syndrome if he had

    A. LDL = 180 and protein/creatinine ratio = 4.

    B. LDL = 129 and protein/creatinine ratio = 3.

    C. LDL = 170 and protein/creatinine ratio = 2.

    D. LDL = 110 and protein/creatinine ratio = 1.

50. Microalbuminuria predicts the development of

    A. Diabetes

    B. Kidney failure

    C. Lupus

    D. Hepatitis B

51. Causes of transient proteinuria include

    A. CHF

    B. Postural hypotension

    C. Dehydration

    D. Diabetes

52. Mr. Fernando has Stage 3 kidney disease and hypertension. Management of hypertension in this patient is complicated by the high risk for

    A. Hypoglycemia

    B. Hyperkalemia

    C. Hyponatremia

    D. Hypercalcemia

53. Systemic kidney disease occurs secondary to which condition?

    A. Diabetes

    B. Hepatitis B

    C. NSAIDs use

    D. All of the above

54. Mrs. Smith, a 70-year-old housewife, has a severe pulsating pain on the left side of her head, which has been present for more than 12 hours with nausea and photophobia; she has some numbness on the left side of her face. Mrs. Smith reports "having this type of headache since she was 18 years old and usually has one headache per month." Mrs. Smith's physical exam is normal. Which of the following types of headache is Mrs. Smith experiencing?

    A. Cluster headache

    B. Episodic tension-type headache

    C. Chronic tension-type headache

    D. Migraine headache

55. Which of the following statements regarding the use of pharmaceuticals for alleviating pain in migraine headache is NOT correct?

A. "NSAIDs have been found to be effective in some migraine patients."

B. "The use of metoclorpramide (Reglan) and phenothiazines enhances the effectiveness of analgesics in the treatment of migraine headaches."

C. "Narcotic analgesics should be used with caution in the treatment of headaches."

D. "Administration of 7 L of oxygen by face mask should be given as early possible after the onset of a migraine headache."

56. Mrs. Webb, a 70-year-old woman, is being treated for chronic tension headaches. She should receive follow-up on a regular basis for all of the following *except*

A. Psychosocial stressors in her life

B. Instructions on various triggers of headaches and how to avoid them

C. Instructions on relaxation and stress-reduction techniques

D. Routine CBC and urinalysis

57. A medication that is appropriate for abortive therapy for an adult client with a migraine is

A. Sumatriptan (Imitrex)

B. Amitriptyline (Elavil)

C. Propanolol

D. Oxycodone

58. Which of the following best describes a tension-type headache?

A. Bilateral, mild to moderate, pressing headache lasting 30 minutes to 7 days.

B. Unilateral, moderate to severe, throbbing headache lasting for 4 to 72 hours, aggravated by routine physical activity, with nausea, vomiting, or both, headache may be preceded by flashing lights.

C. Pounding or dull frontal or occipital pain present when upright and relieved by lying down.

D. More prevalent in men, occurring in attacks of severe unilateral, orbital, super-orbital, or temporal pain, lasting 15 to 180 minutes, with miosis.

59. Which of the following best describes a cluster headache?

    A. Bilateral, mild to moderate, pressing headache lasting 30 minutes to 7 days.

    B. Unilateral, moderate to severe, throbbing headache lasting for 4 to 72 hours, aggravated by routine physical activity, with nausea, vomiting or both, headache may be preceded by flashing lights.

    C. Pounding or dull frontal or occipital pain present when upright and relieved by lying down.

    D. More prevalent in men, occurring in attacks of severe, unilateral orbital, supra-orbital, or temporal pain, lasting 15 to 180 minutes, with miosis.

60. Ms. Donaldson suffers from migraine headaches. In providing teaching to her, it is important to understand that recognized trigger(s) of migraine headache include(s)

    A. Stress, worry, and anxiety

    B. Excessive sleep

    C. Certain foods and alcohol

    D. All of the above

61. The specific nosology or classification for sleep disorders is provided by which organization?

    A. ICD

    B. ICSD

    C. DSM

    D. ACSD

62. Mr. Roth reports a history of sleep problems. In conducting his annual history and physical exam, it is important to remember that the relationship between sleep problems and diabetes is

    A. Causally proven

    B. Predictive

    C. Substantiated but not fully understood

    D. Nonexistent

63. The Actigraph is a sleep assessment instrument that measures

  A. Physical activity

  B. Actions associated with sleepiness

  C. Actions associated with sleep deprivation

  D. Sleep in a qualifiable manner

64. Mr. Roth is diagnosed with a sleep apnea. Which of the following interventions has been found to be the most effective in restoring sleep patterns in this population of patients?

  A. C-PAP machines

  B. Short-acting benzodiazepines

  C. Surgery

  D. SSRIs

65. Delayed sleep-phase syndrome is most associated with which population of patients?

  A. Preschool children

  B. Adolescents

  C. Middle aged adults

  D. Older adults

66. Mr. Paul is returning to you for his PSA test results. In interpreting the results, you know that PSA values more than ___ are highly suspicious for prostate cancer.

  A. 0.4 ng/dl

  B. 0.5 ng/dl

  C. 4.0 ng/dl

  D. 1.0 ng/dl

67. Mr. Brown is returning to you for his PSA test results. In interpreting the results, you know that normal PSA values are generally below

  A. 0.5 ng/dl

  B. 0.75 ng/dl

  C. 1.0 ng/dl

  D. 4.0 ng/dl

68. Mr. Daniels, an 84-year-old male, has just been diagnosed with prostate cancer. Given high rates of overtreatment, the most clinically appropriate prostate cancer management option for men his age with low grade and stage disease and low, stable PSA levels is

    A. Radical prostatectomy

    B. Brachytherapy

    C. External beam radiation

    D. Active surveillance

69. Mr. Johnson, a 90-year-old male, presents to your primary care practice with complaints of erectile dysfunction (ED). In selecting appropriate lab work, you know that the role of decreased testosterone that occurs with aging impacts sexual function

    A. A great deal

    B. Somewhat

    C. Not at all

    D. Minimally

70. Mr. Paul is returning to you for follow-up of ED. In attempting to determine the causative agent for his ED, you know that medications that are believed to influence sexual function among older men include

    A. Calcium channel blockers

    B. Statins

    C. Tricyclic antidepressants

    D. All of the above

71. In recommending treatment for Mr. Green, a 54-year-old male with ED, you consider that the most common form of treatment for male erectile dysfunction is

    A. Oral erectile agents

    B. Surgery

    C. Cavernosal injection therapy

    D. Balloon implants

72. Mr. James, a 73-year-old male, is presenting to your primary care practice with complaints of ED. In conducting his assessment, you know that a major study in Massachusetts confirmed that one of the following is an independent risk factor for ED:

A. Asian ethnicity

B. Single marital status

C. Advanced age

D. Alcohol intake

73. Mr. Johnson is a 49-year-old male who is diagnosed with metabolic syndrome. He is actively trying to lose weight through diet and exercise and taking Lisinopril 40 mg QD and HCTZ 25 mg QD. As the APRN caring for Mr. Johnson, it is very important to also add one of the following categories of medication to his management plan:

A. Oral hypoglycemic

B. Statin

C. Calcium channel blocker

D. Beta blocker

74. Mrs. Payne is a 53-year-old female who is diagnosed with metabolic syndrome. You have provided teaching to her regarding diet and exercise as well as smoking cessation and are managing her blood pressure and cholesterol with medications. Given her high risk for further complications of metabolic syndrome, it is also important to evaluate for and consider adding one of the following categories of medication:

A. Oral hypoglycemic

B. Statin

C. Beta blocker

D. Calcium channel blocker

75. Mr. Paul is a 69-year-old male who is diagnosed with metabolic syndrome. His risk for having an MI with this diagnosis is equivalent to patients with a history of one of the following:

    A. NIDDM

    B. Rheumatoid arthritis

    C. Prior MI

    D. Sickle cell disease

76. Mrs. Williams is presenting to your primary care practice with symptoms consistent with depression. The most important role of the primary care provider related to mental health of patients is

    A. Diagnosis

    B. Prescribing

    C. Referral only

    D. Medication management

77. Mr. Archbold is presenting to your primary care practice for follow-up of multiple medical problems. In conducting his assessment, you choose to administer the CAGE instrument that screens for

    A. Depression

    B. Alcohol

    C. Biopolar disorder

    D. Schizophrenia

78. Mrs. Grace is presenting to your primary care practice with symptoms consistent with depression. In order for her to be properly diagnosed, it is important to know that the DSM-IV-TR diagnosis of depression mandates inclusion of more than ___ depressive symptoms.

    A. 3

    B. 5

    C. 7

    D. 9

79. Mr. Piazza is a 46-year-old male who you are screening for depression. In conducting depression screening in primary care, it is important to remember that 3/4 of patients with depression have the following:

    A. Trouble with authority

    B. Difficulty at work or school

    C. Comorbid disease

    D. Poor family relationships

80. Ms. Gold is presenting to your primary care practice for follow-up of depression. Lifetime treatment of depression is necessary in patients who have had the following number of previous depressive episodes:

    A. 3

    B. 5

    C. 7

    D. 9

81. Mr. Hope is presenting to your primary care practice for follow-up for depression. Referral practices for antidepressant therapy indicates that if no improvement is seen after _____ weeks, therapy should be referred.

    A. 3

    B. 4

    C. 5

    D. 6

82. Mrs. White is presenting to your primary care practice for follow-up of depression. Patients in treatment for depression should visit their health care provider at least every ___ weeks through the first 8 weeks of treatment.

    A. 2

    B. 3

    C. 4

    D. 8

83. Mrs. Naylor is presenting to your primary care practice with symptoms consistent with depression. The most effective treatment plans for depression include one of the following:

    A. Medication

    B. Therapy

    C. Both A and B

    D. Rest and relaxation

84. Mrs. George is an 84-year-old woman newly admitted to your practice. She appears very anxious. In conducting her assessment, it is important to remember that

    A. Anxiety precedes depression in 37% of clinical cases.

    B. Cognitive impairment may be a cause of her anxiety.

    C. Planning for long-term care because this patient is critical.

    D. A cholinesterase inhibitor such as Aricept is very effective in older adults with depression.

85. Which of these statements, if made by the older adult, would be most likely to be an indicator of depression?

    A. "I feel like I have accomplished something today."

    B. "I am just too tired to do anything."

    C. "I would like to visit my daughter."

    D. "My life has had many ups and downs."

86. Mrs. Manual, a 67-year-old female, presents with edema of the DIP joints. With this presentation, the clinician is immediately able to rule out one of the following diagnosis:

    A. Osteoarthritis

    B. Rheumatoid arthritis

    C. Fledgling's disease

    D. Paget's disease

87. In attempting to develop a diagnosis for Ms. Cummings who presents with clinical signs and symptoms of osteoarthritis, it is important to know that classical radiography of osteoarthritis of the knee indicates

    A. Joint space lengthening

    B. Joint space narrowing

    C. Presence of osteophytes

    D. Both B and C

88. Mrs. Wig is presenting to your primary care practice with symptoms consistent with rheumatoid arthritis. Definitive findings for diagnosis of rheumatoid arthritis include

    A. Rheumatoid factor (RF)

    B. Erythrocyte sedimentation rate (ESR)

    C. Absence of joint inflammation

    D. Depends on the joint presentation

89. In conducting a history on Ms. Cummings who presents with clinical signs and symptoms of osteoarthritis, you know that the most common cause of osteoarthritis is

    A. Injury

    B. Paget's disease

    C. Diabetes

    D. Wear and tear

90. Ms. Cummings presents to your primary care practice with synovial cysts. These cysts may occur commonly among patients with

    A. Osteoarthritis

    B. Synarthroses

    C. Hip replacement surgery

    D. Paget's disease

91. Mr. Eli presents with bilateral hand subluxation. This clinical presentation is usually associated with one of the following disorder:

A. Spinal stenosis

B. Osteoarthritis

C. Synovial cysts

D. Rheumatoid arthritis

92. Mr. Nags is an 84-year-old male with c/o numbing and tingling in the fingertips. In attempts to properly classify his condition as primary Raynaud's, you would need to rule out all of the following *except*

A. Cold as a precipitant to the numbness/tingling

B. CREST syndrome

C. The use of ergots

D. Polycythemia

93. Ms. Parker is a 69-year-old woman with a presentation of malar rash, overall body aches and pains and photosensitivity. In order to correctly diagnose systematic lupus erythematosus (SLE), the patient must have ____ criteria occurring simultaneously or serially.

A. 3

B. 4

C. 5

D. All

94. Mr. Paget presents to you for evaluation of a seizure that occurred over the weekend. In selecting the most important diagnostics for this presentation, it is important to know that the most common site of seizures is

A. Cerebellum

B. Frontal lobe

C. Temporal lobe

D. Parietal lobe

95. Mrs. Datry is a 59-year-old patient newly diagnosed with epilepsy. Patient education for patients with epilepsy must include

    A. Medications

    B. Avoidance of precipitants to seizure

    C. Safety issues (no climbing, driving, swimming alone, etc.)

    D. All of the above

96. A 69-year-old patient is admitted with generalized seizures and is receiving phenytoin (Dilantin) and Phenobarbital. Phenytoin levels are monitored. Which of the following laboratory values for phenytoin is within the therapeutic level?

    A. 15 ug/ml

    B. 31 ug/ml

    C. 51 ug/ml

    D. 71 ug/ml

97. Which of the following characterizes status epileptics?

    A. Akinetic movements

    B. Monoclonic movements

    C. Generalized seizure activity without regaining consciousness

    D. Brief loss of contact with the environment

98. When a patient suddenly appears to be having a seizure, the clinician would

    A. Initiate airway, breathing, and circulation

    B. Administer oxygen via nasal route as needed

    C. Have suction available and place patient on his or her side

    D. All of the above

99. Diagnostic studies to diagnose new onset epilepsy accurately may include

    A. EEG

    B. CT/MRI to identify brain lesions

    C. Neuropsychologic evaluation

    D. All of the above

100. Mrs. Blackmon presents with a raised spot on her arm measuring more than 5 mm. You know that this is called a

    A. Macule

    B. Papule

    C. Nodule

    D. Patch

101. Mr. Jordan is diagnosed with atopic dermatitis (AD). In monitoring his progress with this disorder, it is important to remember that the distribution of AD

    A. Remains stable over time

    B. Changes throughout the lifespan

    C. Is always the same

    D. Depends upon exposure

102. Mr. Hart is presenting to the primary care practice with signs and symptoms of syncope. For a true diagnosis of syncope to be determined, which of the following must be present?

    A. Shortness of breath on exertion

    B. Headache

    C. Dizziness

    D. Loss of consciousness

103. Mr. Hart continues to complain of dizziness. In trying to determine the differentials associated with this complaint, you know that the most common differentials associated with vertigo include

    A. Peripheral neuropathy

    B. Diabetes

    C. Meniere's disease

    D. Rheumatoid arthritis (RA)

104. Mr. Hart continues to complain of dizziness. In trying to determine the differentials associated with this complaint, you know that the most common differentials associated with *disequilibrium* include

    A. Peripheral neuropathy

    B. Diabetes

    C. Meniere's disease

    D. Anemia

105. Mr. Hart continues to complain of dizziness. In trying to determine the differentials associated with this complaint, you know that the most common differentials associated with *syncope* include

    A. Peripheral neuropathy

    B. Diabetes

    C. Meniere's disease

    D. Rheumatoid arthritis (RA)

106. Medications associated with dizziness include one of the following:

    A. Antihypertensives

    B. Narcotics

    C. Benzodiazepines

    D. All of the above

107. Mr. Sand presents with signs and symptoms of contact dermatitis. The most important history question to ask patients who present with contact dermatitis is

  A. How long have you had it?

  B. What have you done for it?

  C. What is your occupation?

  D. Do you use sun block?

108. Mrs. Patterson presents with complaints of vertigo. A hallmark of benign positional vertigo is that

  A. It only occurs when the client is supine

  B. It usually occurs after a viral illness

  C. The sensation of vertigo remains as long as the position is maintained

  D. The symptoms occur with positional changes and last for a few minutes

109. Mr. Radner has multiple sclerosis (MS). In classifying the progression of disability, you explain that the most common type of disease is

  A. Relapsing–remitting

  B. Secondary–progressive

  C. Primary–progressive

  D. Progressive–relapsing

110. In the case of Mr. Potter, a 34-year-old man, undergoing a diagnostic work-up for MS, it is important to assess for which of the most commonly presenting sensory symptoms for MS?

  A. Pain

  B. Numbness and tingling in extremities

  C. Burning in hands and feet

  D. Constriction feelings in neck

111. Mr. Heath presents to the clinic with various neurological complaints including a deficiency in his sense of smell. After ruling out ENT causes, you know that the most common neurological disorder associated with loss of smell sensation is

    A. Multiple sclerosis (MS)

    B. Amyotrophic lateral sclerosis (ALS)

    C. Brain tumor

    D. Parkinson's disease (PD)

112. Mr. Lower's treatment for MS includes a specified medication regime. In planning his care, it is important to remember that all medications for MS must be administered

    A. By mouth

    B. Through injectable routes

    C. Sublingually

    D. Via suppository

113. Mr. Flower, a patient with MS, presents with a self-diagnosed relapse of MS. In order to be classified as a true relapse, symptoms must be impeding function for _____ hours.

    A. 6

    B. 12

    C. 24

    D. 48

114. Mr. Ingersoll is recently diagnosed with amyotrophic lateral sclerosis (ALS). In discussing medication treatment with him, you know that the only FDA approved medication for ALS is _____.

    A. Tysabri (natalizumab)

    B. Novantrone

    C. Copaxone (glatiramer)

    D. Riluzole (rilutek)

115. Mrs. L is an 84-year-old woman who takes an opioid for chronic non-malignant pain. She does not like to take pills and usually waits until her pain is excruciating before doing so. You are trying to explain why it is more beneficial for her to take the medication regularly than when her pain is extreme. Which of the following is true?

    A. She will not become dependent on the medication because it is medically necessary.

    B. Keeping the pain at a lower level will improve effectiveness of the medication.

    C. If she does not use the medication regularly, her pain will become more severe over time.

    D. The pain is damaging her nervous system. If she does not control it, she will lose some nervous system function.

116. Mrs. F has chronic pain related to arthritis. She has recently displayed drug seeking behaviors such as hoarding her pills and becoming anxious about getting refills. As the primary care provider for Mrs. F, you are most concerned about

    A. Addiction

    B. Poor pain control

    C. Polypharmacy

    D. Dementia

117. An older woman who suffers from chronic back pain from osteoporosis calls your office to say that her pain has suddenly increased today and she wants a stronger medicine to be phoned into her pharmacy. She is currently taking a long acting opioid. The best approach to treating her is to

    A. Add acetaminophen to her regimen and see her tomorrow

    B. Make no medication changes, but schedule a psychological evaluation as soon as possible.

    C. Prescribe a higher dosage of medicine she is currently taking and squeeze her in tomorrow.

    D. Squeeze her into your schedule today before making any medication changes.

118. A caretaker brings a nonverbal, severely retarded 50-year-old woman into the clinic who she believes to be in pain. Clinical findings to support this presentation include

   A. Low blood pressure

   B. Bradycardia

   C. Restlessness

   D. Somnolence

119. For which of the following patients would a tricyclic antidepressant be most appropriate for pain management?

   A. 55-year-old man with 10 year history of type 2 diabetes with burning foot pain for 1 year.

   B. 55-year-old man with 3 week history of low back pain.

   C. 55-year-old man with 5 year history of chronic back pain and depression, currently taking an SSRI.

   D. 55-year-old man 2 days post shoulder surgery.

120. Mr. Parkson is recently diagnosed with back pain for which he is being treated with opioids. You think he may be experiencing signs/symptoms of pseudoaddiction which is best defined as

   A. A primary, chronic, neurobiological disease characterized by impaired control over drug use.

   B. A state of adaptation that is manifested by a specific withdrawal syndrome that is produced by an abrupt cessation of a drug.

   C. A pattern of drug seeking behavior because the patient is receiving inadequate pain management.

   D. A pain state where more than one pain medication is needed to control the pain.

121. Mrs. Packer has been diagnosed with congestive heart failure (CHF). Cardinal manifestations of heart failure that should consistently be assessed include

   A. Dyspnea, fatigue, and fluid retention

   B. Fever, fatigue, and dyspnea

   C. Dyspnea, ankle edema, and chest pain

   D. Elevated leukocytes, dyspnea, and fluid retention

122. Which least invasive diagnostic study would be most beneficial in assessing left ventricular ejection fraction in Mrs. Packer, a patient diagnosed with CHF?

    A. Cardiac catheterization

    B. Dual isotope stress test

    C. Electrocardiogram

    D. Chest x-ray

123. Mrs. Joran is an elderly patient with a diagnosis of left-sided CHF. The nurse practitioner would identify what common condition frequently associated with this diagnosis?

    A. History or peripheral vascular disease

    B. History of poorly treated hypertension

    C. Current treatment for ventricular dysrhythmias

    D. History of COPD

124. Mr. Schwartz has been diagnosed with CHF. Which of the following is most essential in the prevention of development and/or progression of heart failure?

    A. Exercise

    B. Dietary restriction of sodium

    C. Rigorous management of hypertension

    D. Adherence to pharmacological regime

125. Mrs. Paulhus has been diagnosed with CHF. Risk factors for developing CHF include all the following, *except*

    A. Diabetes

    B. Older age

    C. Female gender

    D. Greater body mass index

126. Mr. Kline has been diagnosed with left-sided CHF. The principle hallmark of patients with systolic dysfunction related to CHF is

   A. Increased resistance to ventricular filling

   B. Loss of myocardial relaxation

   C. Reduced ejection fraction

   D. Valvular dysfunction

127. Ms. Chin is a 79-year-old woman who presents to the family practice clinic for the first time. Which of the following red flag symptoms might Ms. Chin exhibit that would most likely lead you to suspect that she is a victim of domestic violence?

   A. Somatic complaints without diagnosis

   B. Hyperlipidemia

   C. Obesity

   D. Vaginal discharge

128. In screening Ms. Chin for domestic violence, a good framing statement may be

   A. You look like you are a typical victim of abuse.

   B. Unfortunately, violence often plays a role in many relationships.

   C. Do you have any questions or concerns about domestic violence?

   D. What brings you in today?

129. Ms. Fly is a 69-year-old woman who presents to the family practice clinic for the first time. Consistent with evidence about the prevalence of domestic violence, you know that you must screen for domestic violence

   A. At all patient encounters

   B. At visits for complete physical exams

   C. Only when the patient admits to being a victim

   D. When signs and symptoms of domestic violence are suspected

130. During Ms. Chin's second visit to the family practice clinic for diabetic teaching, she is accompanied by her partner. Which partner behavior is most consistent with domestic violence?

    A. Partner is supportive and asks appropriate questions

    B. Partner asks if the practitioner knows how the wife acquired diabetes

    C. Partner answers questions for the patient and will not leave patient unattended

    D. Partner exchanges jokes with patient about not being able to eat at the family bakery

131. Ms. Appleton accidentally cut her eye lid with a knife while carving a pumpkin with her grandchildren last weekend. The wound is approximately 3 cm with clean approximated edges. The most appropriate material with which to close the wound is

    A. Skin adhesives

    B. Staples

    C. Sutures

    D. Steri-strips

132. Mrs. Appleton in the previous question cannot recall when she had her last tetanus shot, but believes it may have been about 6 years ago when she entered graduate school. How would you proceed in regards to ensuring adequate immunization against tetanus?

    A. She does not need a tetanus booster as she had one within the last 6 years.

    B. She does not need a tetanus booster as she has had multiple boosters since initial immunization during childhood.

    C. Administer a tetanus booster, as she is unclear as to when her last booster was administered.

    D. She does not need a tetanus booster, as this is a clean wound.

133. Which of the following descriptions of a referral and a consultation is true?

    A. A consultation is officially telephoned in by your office and indicates a need for specialized management and treatment.

    B. A referral is a request that another provider accept ongoing treatment responsibility for a patient needing specialized care.

    C. A consultation may occur informally but does indicate a change of responsibility for patient management.

    D. A consultation requires the client to be sent to another health care provider for a more in-depth evaluation by a specialist who will assume primary responsibility for this patient's management.

134. The following organization develops the competencies of care which NPs must be able to demonstrate upon graduation of their NP program:

    A. American College of Nurse Practitioner Association

    B. International Society of Nurse Practitioners

    C. American Academy of Nurse Practitioner Association

    D. National Organization of Nurse Practitioner Faculties

135. Zero-based budgeting refers to a budgeting system that

    A. Accounts for unexpected budget variances.

    B. Accounts for expected budget variances only

    C. Justifies each budget on its own merits, not on the basis of the previous period's budget

    D. Justifies each budget based on the previous period's budget

136. Credentialing of nurse practitioners means that

    A. An individual is permitted to practice advanced practice nursing

    B. The practitioner has met certain criteria through licensure, certification, and education

    C. An individual has completed a program of study

    D. An individual has prescriptive authority

137. The purpose of the ANA's Scope and Standards of Family Nursing Practice is to

    A. Define the role and actions for the NP

    B. Establish the legal authority for the prescription of medications

    C. Define the legal statutes of the role of the FNP

    D. Define the differences between the physician role and the NP role

138. The major barriers to full implementation of an autonomous role for APRNs in primary care include

    A. The need for medical specialists because of rapidly changing technologies

    B. The increasingly complex health problems of vulnerable populations

    C. Prescriptive authority, scope of practice, and reimbursement

    D. Managed care organizations' views of APRNs

139. A community has an unusual high incidence of obesity and drug use among the older adult population. The Community Health Center nurse practitioners decide to address this problem, in part, by modifying the environment and strengthening the capacities of families to prevent further complications for the individuals diagnosed with diabetes and substance abuse. This is an example of

    A. Primary prevention

    B. Secondary prevention

    C. Tertiary prevention

    D. Protective factorial protection

140. What are the three basic components of an NP-client relationship?

    1. Prescriptive and nonprescriptive therapeutics

    2. Promoting trust

    3. Maintaining professional boundaries

    4. Using therapeutic communication

    A. 1, 2, 4

    B. 2, 3

    C. 2, 3, 4

    D. 1, 3, 4

141. You are preparing to perform a health history on Mr. P in the clinic for the first time. You understand that the purpose of a health history is to

    A. Analyze data that has already been collected.

    B. Review any past collaborative problems.

    C. Provide subjective data for the health assessment.

    D. Consult with the client's family members.

142. Scott P. is preparing to conduct a health history on a 60-year-old man as part of his insurance physical. The primary purpose of a health assessment is to

    A. Gather information to identify real and potential diagnoses and interventions.

    B. Gather data about a person's health.

    C. Identify patterns of functioning that conform to or deviate from norms.

    D. Collect data related to psychosocial symptoms.

143. Mrs. Crotwell has been hospitalized with a medical diagnosis of osteoporosis and compression fracture of the lumbar spine. She complains of lower back pain while ambulating. Based on this data, your documentation should include

    A. The amount ambulated and the complaint of pain

    B. The amount ambulated only

    C. The complaint of pain only

    D. None of the above; this is routine nursing care

144. You are required to take a health history on an older adult health clinic. Select the best description of "review of systems" as part of this health history.

    A. The evaluation of the past and present health state of each body system

    B. A documentation of the problem as described by the patient

    C. The recording of the objective findings of the practitioner

    D. A statement that describes the overall health state of the patient

145. The head and neck exam is unique in which it:

    A. Is essential in detecting cancer

    B. Is amenable to examination without violation of privacy

    C. Only requires the skills of palpation

    D. Only requires the skills of inspection

146. Forced inspiration commands the use of accessory _____ muscles to lift the sternum and rib cage.

    A. Sternocleidomastoid

    B. Neck

    C. Gluteus maximus

    D. Vastus lateralis

147. Wheezes are most consistent with which of the following respiratory condition?

    A. Pneumonia

    B. Upper airway obstruction

    C. Asthma

    D. Lung cancer

148. Vesicular lung sounds may be heard in

    A. Most of the lungs

    B. Bronchovesicular spaces

    C. Over the trachea

    D. In the parenchyma

149. Which coronary vessels bring freshly oxygenated blood to the left side of the heart?

    A. Superior vena cava

    B. Inferior vena cava

    C. Pulmonary artery

    D. Pulmonary veins

150. Right-sided heart failure is usually manifested by which of the following symptoms?

    A. Respiratory wheezes

    B. Jugular vein constriction

    C. Respiratory crackles

    D. Peripheral edema

151. If bruits or thrills are assessed in carotid arteries, the most appropriate follow-up test would be which of the following?

    A. Magnetic resonance imaging (MRI)

    B. Carotid x-ray

    C. Carotid ultrasound

    D. EKG

152. What is the criterion for visual acuity using the Snellen eye test?

    A. Smallest line of print that is read correctly

    B. Line of print where the patient started reading the chart

    C. Size of the largest printed letters read from the chart

    D. Speed at which the printed letters are read correctly

153. When testing visual fields, where should the examiner be positioned?

    A. Sitting on the side of the patient, facing the same direction as the patient

    B. Sitting on the side of the patient, facing the patient

    C. Sitting directly behind the patient, with hands facing the patient

    D. Standing directly in front of the patient, facing the patient

154. The examiner holds up wiggling fingers lateral to the patient's ears, on both sides, simultaneously. At the beginning of the test, on what should the patient keep her eyes fixed?

    A. Examiner's fingers

    B. Examiner's eyes

    C. Central place on the wall

    D. Examining light

155. When a lightly vibrating tuning fork is placed on top of the head and the sound is heard in the left ear only, this reveals abnormal lateralization of sound. What is the name of this test?

    A. Rinne test

    B. Allen test

    C. Weber test

    D. Pneumatic test

156. The examiner places a lightly vibrating tuning fork on the mastoid bone behind the ear and level with the canal. When the patient can no longer hear the sound, the tuning fork is moved quickly to the ear canal to determine if the sound can be heard again. What is the principle behind this test?

    A. In normal hearing, vibrations are heard longer than felt

    B. In normal hearing, vibrations are felt longer than sound

    C. In normal hearing, sound is heard longer through air than bone

    D. In normal hearing, sound is heard longer through bone than air

157. Which of the following is a charting example that can be found under the ROS?

    A. Denies blurred vision, eye pain, or ear pain

    B. PERRLA, EOMI, fundi-sharp bilaterally w/o AV nicking or hemorrhages

    C. +DM 2 × 15 years, + renal insufficiency × 2 years, −HTN

    D. +tonsillectomy in 1980

158. On an annual health history for a 55-year-old patient, which of the following questions would be most appropriate to ask when collecting information pertaining to routine health maintenance?

    A. Have you ever had a colonoscopy?

    B. Do you take any herbal supplements?

    C. Do you have a history of hypertension?

    D. Have you ever been hospitalized?

159. Which of the following techniques is a critical factor with every physical exam and should be performed initially and throughout the exam?

A. Palpation

B. Auscultation

C. Percussion

D. Inspection

160. You are assessing the carotid arteries. You find a carotid bruit. What does this mean?

A. The patient has increased blood circulation to the head

B. The artery is probably stenotic or atherosclerotic

C. The patient also has an S3 heart sound

D. The artery is patent but thin walled

161. Mrs. Chancey is a 69-year-old Caucasian female who has agreed to take a DEXA assessment to determine her bone density. In interpreting the results, you know that normal bone T-scores are

A. T-score between −1 and −2.5

B. T-score better than −1

C. T-score less than −2.5

D. T-score above −2.5

162. Mr. Golden is an 84-year-old man who is entering the hospital for treatment of pneumonia. In counseling him before admission, you know that the primary source of payment for older adult health care is

A. Medicare

B. Medicaid

C. Private insurance

D. Medigap

163. GNP's role in quality improvement projects may include which of the following?

    A. Identifying standards of care

    B. Articulate a trend in patient care problems

    C. Select the best evidence and implementing it into clinical practice

    D. All of the above

164. A GNP is working on a research study that is testing an oral medication on wound healing of all patients with wounds in a long-term care facility over a 1-year period of time. How would you describe the study design used in this case?

    A. Descriptive, cross sectional

    B. Experimental, longitudinal

    C. Quasi experimental, longitudinal

    D. Experimental, cross sectional

165. If the GNP was interested in developing an instrument to measure the subtle symptoms of diabetes exhibited by subjects in this study and wanted to test it to make sure it measured what it was supposed to measure, what would she be testing for?

    A. Reliability

    B. Velocity

    C. Heterogeneity

    D. Validity

Answers

CHAPTER 3

1. B
2. C
3. C
4. C
5. A
6. B
7. A
8. C
9. A
10. B
11. B
12. B
13. B
14. B
15. C

CHAPTER 4

1. C
2. A
3. B
4. D
5. C
6. D
7. D
8. B
9. A
10. D
11. B
12. C
13. D
14. A
15. C

CHAPTER 5

1. B
2. C
3. D
4. A
5. B
6. C
7. D
8. A
9. B
10. A
11. D
12. B
13. C
14. A
15. C
16. C
17. B
18. A
19. A
20. C
21. A
22. B
23. C
24. A
25. D
26. A
27. A
28. B
29. D
30. C
31. D
32. B

33. C
34. B
35. A
36. B
37. C
38. B
39. C
40. B

CHAPTER 6

1. A
2. C
3. D
4. A
5. B
6. C
7. A
8. B
9. A
10. C
11. B
12. A
13. D
14. C
15. A

CHAPTER 7

1. B
2. D
3. A
4. D
5. A
6. B

7. C
8. A
9. D
10. D
11. B
12. A
13. B
14. B
15. B

CHAPTER 8

1. D
2. D
3. C
4. B
5. D
6. A
7. C
8. C
9. C
10. D
11. B
12. D
13. A
14. B
15. A

QUESTION BANK

1. C
2. D
3. B
4. D
5. A
6. B
7. C
8. C
9. B
10. B
11. B
12. C
13. C
14. A

15. C
16. D
17. C
18. B
19. A
20. B
21. A
22. D
23. A
24. C
25. C
26. C
27. D
28. C
29. B
30. C
31. A
32. C
33. A
34. B
35. C
36. C
37. A
38. B
39. B
40. C
41. A
42. D
43. B
44. C
45. A
46. D
47. B
48. B
49. D
50. B
51. A
52. B
53. D
54. D
55. D
56. D
57. A

58. A
59. D
60. D
61. B
62. C
63. A
64. A
65. B
66. C
67. C
68. D
69. D
70. D
71. A
72. C
73. B
74. A
75. C
76. A
77. B
78. B
79. C
80. A
81. B
82. A
83. C
84. A
85. B
86. B
87. D
88. D
89. D
90. A
91. D
92. A
93. B
94. C
95. D
96. A
97. C
98. D
99. D
100. C

101. B	**123.** B	**145.** B
102. D	**124.** C	**146.** A
103. C	**125.** C	**147.** C
104. C	**126.** C	**148.** A
105. B	**127.** A	**149.** D
106. D	**128.** B	**150.** D
107. C	**129.** A	**151.** C
108. D	**130.** C	**152.** A
109. A	**131.** C	**153.** D
110. B	**132.** C	**154.** B
111. C	**133.** B	**155.** C
112. B	**134.** D	**156.** C
113. C	**135.** C	**157.** A
114. D	**136.** B	**158.** A
115. B	**137.** A	**159.** D
116. B	**138.** C	**160.** B
117. D	**139.** C	**161.** B
118. C	**140.** C	**162.** A
119. A	**141.** C	**163.** D
120. C	**142.** A	**164.** C
121. A	**143.** A	**165.** D
122. B	**144.** A	

Index